T0074007

Sports and Traumatology

Series Editor

Philippe Landreau
Doha, Qatar

As more and more people are getting involved in sports, even the elderly, sports traumatology has become a recognized medical specialty. In sports exercises, every joint and every anatomical region can become the location of a traumatic injury: an acute trauma, a series of repeated microtraumas or even an overuse pathology. Different sports activities may produce different and specific traumas in the same anatomical region. The aim of the book series 'Sports and Traumatology' is to present in each book a description of the state of the art on treating the broad range of lesions and the mechanisms in sports activities that cause them. Sports physicians, surgeons, rehabilitation specialists and physiotherapists will find books that address their daily clinical and therapeutic concerns.

More information about this series at http://www.springer.com/series/8671

Herbert Schoenhuber • Andrea Panzeri
Simone Porcelli

Editors

Alpine Skiing Injuries

Prevention and Management

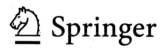 Springer

Editors
Herbert Schoenhuber
IRCCS Galeazzi Orthopaedics Institute
Milan, Milano, Italy

President Medical Committee
Winter Sport Italian Federation
Milan, Italy

Andrea Panzeri
IRCCS Galeazzi Orthopaedics Institute
Milan, Milano, Italy

Vice President Medical Committee
Winter Sport Italian Federation
Milan, Italy

Simone Porcelli
National Research Council
Milan, Milano, Italy

Member Medical Committee
Winter Sport Italian Federation
Milan, Italy

ISSN 2105-0759   ISSN 2105-0538   (electronic)
Sports and Traumatology
ISBN 978-3-319-61354-3   ISBN 978-3-319-61355-0   (eBook)
https://doi.org/10.1007/978-3-319-61355-0

Library of Congress Control Number: 2017960966

Printed on acid-free paper

This Springer imprint is published by Springer Nature
The registered company is Springer International Publishing AG
The registered company address is: Gewerbestrasse 11, 6330 Cham, Switzerland

Preface

Ski, sport and mountain.

The passion for winter sports disciplines has always been with me from the beginning of my medical career.

I have worked in FISI (Italian Winter Sports Federation) for almost 30 years and in the Medical Committee of the FIS (International Ski Federation) for almost 20 years. During this period I lived many experiences: victories, defeats, struggles and goals.

I worked, and I'm still working, with a lot of professionals in different disciplines that I consider my great teachers and friends.

In this continuous learning experience, I have taken part in numerous projects for the development of safety in skiing and I have fought many battles for safety on the front line.

All this always driven by love for sport and for medicine.

Working alongside numerous professionals and athletes has been an unforgettable and unique experience that made me grow up both professionally and personally.

This book shows a part of the great work that FISI does annually with athletes, in its big family.

Milan, Italy   Herbert Schoenhuber

Contents

1   **Biomechanics of Alpine Skiing**   1
Alberto E. Minetti

2   **Physiology of Alpine Skiing**   9
Simone Porcelli and Marco Zancanaro

3   **Training and Testing for Elite Skiers**   17
Roberto Manzoni and Andrea Viano

4   **Epidemiology of Alpine Skiing Injuries**   31
Marco Freschi

5   **Concussion in Alpine Ski**   41
Zefferino Rossini, Francesco Costa, Alessandro Ortolina,
Massimo Tomei, Maurizio Fornari, and Valentina Re

6   **Traumatic Dislocation and Fractures**   57
Andrea Panzeri, Paolo Capitani, Gabriele Thiébat,
and Herbert Schoenhuber

7   **Overuse Injuries in Alpine Skiers**   77
Gabriele Thiébat, Andrea Panzeri, Paolo Capitani,
and Herbert Schoenhuber

8   **Prevention of Overuse Injuries in Alpine Skiers**   83
Roberto Manzoni, Enea Bortoluz, and Alberto Sugliano

9   **Musculoskeletal Disorders Among Elite Alpine Skiing Racers**   91
Gianluca Melegati

10 **Return to Elite Alpine Sports Activity After Injury**   103
Roberto Manzoni, Enea Bortoluz, and Alberto Sugliano

11   Role of Ski Equipment on Injury Rate 113
Paolo Capitani, Gabriele Thiébat, Andrea Panzeri, and Herbert
Schoenhuber

12   Respiratory System Illness and Hypoxia 123
Manuela Bartesaghi and Giuseppe Miserocchi

Chapter 1
Biomechanics of Alpine Skiing

Alberto E. Minetti

Abstract Understanding the biomechanics of Alpine skiing is fundamental to the design of training protocols, to identify the metabolic burden of athletes and to help preventing traumas. Despite the apparent simplicity of the overall mechanics related to a descent with skiis, the scientific community is still uncertain about the role of muscle contraction in controlling the trajectory on the snow and about the partitioning between force and skill in determining the performance outcome. Generally speaking, skiers increase their body energy (in terms of potential energy) by taking the cable car up to the mountain top; then, to reach the bottom of the track, all that energy needs to be dissipated (as heat). There are just three dissipators involved: snow, air and muscles. If muscles play a major role in transforming potential energy into heat, they need to contract eccentrically, and athletes should be mostly trained in that respect. Conversely, if snow (and its displacement) is responsible for most of the slowdown of the skier, it would be advisable for racers to be trained to generate force both concentrically and eccentrically, with a deeper focus on controlling the fast and intense alternation of the two muscle conditions (a sort of 'intensively perturbed isometric contraction'). This chapter starts from constraints from physics and, through experimental data, tries to shed light on this, still debated topic.

1.1 Introduction

It is very likely that the first seed towards the development and diffusion of Alpine ski appeared a few thousand years BCE (Before Common Era) in geographical areas where no Alps exist and most of the terrain is rather plain. Skiis were invented and intensively used by Laps, Siberian and Scandinavian peoples to transverse long distances during the harsh winter season, where moving without external aids would have resulted in a tiring, slow and uneconomical sinking progression in the

A.E. Minetti
Faculty of Medicine, Laboratory of Locomotion Physiomechanics,
Department of Pathophysiology and Transplantation, University of Milan, Milan, Italy
e-mail: alberto.minetti@unimi.it

© Springer International Publishing AG 2018
H. Schoenhuber et al. (eds.), *Alpine Skiing Injuries*, Sports and Traumatology,
https://doi.org/10.1007/978-3-319-61355-0_1

1

snow. But what we now call cross country skiing included, even at those times, some downhill parts of the track where it was less important to push on the ski poles, but the trajectory still needed to be accurately controlled. For this reason, some of the skiis still visible in Scandinavian Museums show a set of parallel grooves underneath [1].

Modern Alpine skiing is the result of the last 150 years slow convergence towards the best methodology to move along steep snow descents. This process started by including a sort of alpenstock, which was soon duplicated resulting in the actual pair of ski poles. Despite of the crucial use of upper limbs for balancing and unloading body weight at the ski/snow interface, most of the physiological and biomechanical attention so far was focused on the lower limb and trunk muscles which contrast the tendency of the body structure to collapse in landing after jumps and during fast turns. An apparently simple question about how muscles work in Alpine skiing is still a matter of debate. Activated muscles, depending on the load, can develop force and shorten (positive mechanical work), lengthen (negative work) or remain at his length (zero work).

Although this chapter could have had considered other important biomechanical aspects, as the biomechanics of injuries in skiing, the relevance of answering that ancestral question, with the idea that muscles appropriately trained to face their actual usage, seemed fundamental also for injury prevention.

1.2   Physics of Alpine Skiing

Environmental constraints in Alpine ski are a downhill slope, the presence of snow/ice and the effects of air on the skier's motion.

Despite of some flat, or even slightly uphill, portions of the track, the trajectory can be assimilated to a monotonic descent from a higher to a lower altitude level. This involves the inevitable transformation of body potential energy (PE = $m \cdot g \cdot \Delta h$, where m is mass, g is gravity and Δh is the altitude difference) into other forms of energy as kinetic energy and heat. The first form is conservative and mostly desired, as the skier gains speed and all efforts go to maximise it (racing) or to reach a leisure level. In each case, the speed needs to be controlled, because geometric characteristics of the track (bumps and turns, for instance) could lead to dangerous accelerations and uncontrolled landing and conduct. An excessive speed increase (high kinetic energy, KE = $1/2\ m \cdot v^2$, where v is skier's speed) is very difficult to control, and its sudden dissipation, through high decelerations, would impact on the integrity of body structures and organs.

PE is also partly converted into heat for two reasons: snow friction and air drag. Both transformations are dissipative, as the skier cannot in any way transform heat back into PE (or KE). Air friction causes air drag, which is directed in the same direction of the motion but with an opposite versus. It depends on the speed squared, and the other crucial determinants are the frontal area of the subject and its 3D shape. The decelerating effect thus relies on the skier posture and garment fabric, which are optimised in racing. Snow friction is somehow a desired effect, as it is partly controlled by the skiers during turns in the attempt to closely follow the imposed trajectory (racing) and to avoid excessive speed gain (leisure skiing). Such a dissipative transformation is a challenge for researchers as it relies on snow/ski interactions, which is a very complex topic. Snow conditions can vary a lot, mainly depending on air temperature, pressure, wind and humidity. Also snowfall history and track conditioning can affect the measured friction. On the other hand, skiis underwent huge technological developments in the last 100 years, with the recent introduction of carved skiis. Ski width, length, carving radius and the chosen material for blades and bottom (and its waxing) greatly affect the interaction with the snow. However, if those determinants make static and dynamic friction being (barely) measurable on straight parts of the track, this becomes a real challenge when analysing turns, where ski/snow contact area and sidecut vary according to speed, carved/turn radius, skidding, body leaning and trajectory angle with respect to the (maximum) terrain slope. All these parameters affect the creation of the water film between the ski and the snow, which decreases the overall friction and makes PE to KE transformation, namely, skiing, possible.

As the skier starts and ends his/her descent at zero speed, we can expect that all the previously cumulated PE (by cable car), due to the altitude difference, has to be dissipated to heat. A decrease in mechanical energy is called negative work, while increase is (positive) work. Skiing involves positive work done by gravity (as movement occurs in the same direction and versus of the force) and snow; air and other actuators (see below) perform negative work by resisting the body acceleration downward (also hitting gates during races and bending skiis at mid-turn correspond to some negative work, adding to body deceleration). Obviously, the amount of positive and negative works has to be equal at the end of a descent.

As already mentioned, the role of other (biological) 'actuators', namely, muscles, in actively slowing down body motion has been a matter of debate for quite a long time. We will try to address this point in the next section. It is true, though, that the mystery is not just imputable to the lack of biomechanical research, as ski/snow friction remains very difficult to be reliably assessed.

An enlightening question should be: how much is the minimum amount of 'active negative work' necessary to descend on skiis? A possible answer is that snow plough (introduced as the 'Arlberg technique' by Hannes Schneider in 1910) can be performed by a rigid mechanical model with no extra negative work (with respect to the ones made by air and snow friction). The objection that snowplough is not exactly skiing, a mechanical passive skier model, produced by Helmut Gottschlich and Hans Zehetmayer in 1968 (https://www.youtube.com/watch?v=cfEzIcFTq_o, starting at 9:40), showed that it is possible to produce 'slalom-like' descents with zero extra negative work.

A final, additional question for biomechanists is: particularly during races, could muscle activity provide positive work to further (with respect to PE transformation, and some elastic energy release from ski shape restoring after bending) increase skier's speed (KE)? If a complete mechanical energy balance of skiing could be measured, any increase in total body energy (TE = PE + KE) during the descent could be interpreted as an active muscle production of positive work.

1.3   Biomechanics of Alpine Skiing

Body constraints in Alpine ski are (a) a multi-segment skeleton mainly favouring sagittal movements but with many degrees of freedom of its joints; (b) actuators (muscles) that exert force only directed towards their centre, whether they shorten, lengthen or act isometrically; and (c) the neuromuscular control, which is affected by the number of muscles involved, by the amount of the generated force and by the timing between signal detection and useful reaction. The result is a far-from-rigid body in the need of stiffening action of agonist and antagonist muscles to cope with the maintenance of posture and, in skiing, with the continuous perturbation of its geometry due to ground reaction forces generated to counteract gravity (during landing) and centripetal acceleration (during turns).

When we stand, our muscles perform almost isometrically, to fix posture and balancing throughout micro-adjustments. An isometric activity involves no mechanical work (as there is no movement of muscle insertions), but the force is generated at the cost of ATP breakdown, thus with some metabolic consumption [2]. During skiing such a fixative function is certainly higher than in standing, as muscles need to often contrast a force much higher than body weight (during landing and turns), with moment arms of the more flexed joints that amplify the force muscles have to generate.

According to the concepts introduced in the previous paragraphs, downhill skiing with turns could be sustained just by stiffening our joints (isometric contractions) and let our body behaving as the quoted passive mechanical model. But, skiing implies choosing the right trajectory, interactively contrasting unexpected terrain/snow unevenness and, in racing, trying to maintain the speed as high as possible. Those goals can be achieved only if muscles act both as motors (positive work) and dumpers (negative work), i.e. when they generate force during shortening and lengthening, respectively.

The question, then, is not about the ratio between the total amount of shortening and of lengthening during a descent, which by definition has to be 1, but it deals with the overall amount of useful force for braking (negative work) and the one for increasing body mechanical energy (positive work). Despite a couple of attempts to provide those measurements in the literature [3], a complete picture of them, which could deeply influence the training regime designed for athletes, is still lacking. Also, the three specialities of Alpine ski should be separately investigated as the partitioning and type of turns and straight portions of the track, not to mention the speed, vary considerably among slalom, giant slalom, super-G and downhill ski. What we know for sure about those race variations is that extra (muscle-driven) negative work, if measured, will be the prevalent form and very likely much higher than the extra positive one, if any.

To quantitatively assess muscle activity in skiing, complex experimental proto-col and setup are required: subjects should wear a high spatial/temporal resolution GNSS device (capable of sampling at high frequency the signal coming GPS, GLONASS and Galileo satellite constellations) also sensing barometric altitude, to accurately track body position in 3D, electromyographic (EMG) electrodes posi-tioned on the principal postural and propulsive muscles of the trunk/limbs, electro-goniometers located on the involved joints and a data logger that collect all these data synchronously (with the atomic time provided by GNSS).

Additional information includes a high-resolution 3D planimetry (GIS files) of the terrain where ski tracks have been designed, a static 2D camera with high optical magnification and, possibly, a drone following the skier downhill to capture the body segment motion from a close distance. We recently arranged a similar experi-mental session in Cervinia [4]. Post-processing of the sampled data dealt with phys-ics first and biomechanics later. 3D body position, sampled at 10 Hz, allowed to obtain the skier's instantaneous speed and the radius of each turn (which could be compared to the ski sidecut). Together with position on the 3D terrain planimetry and two crucial angles (the maximum slope around the point of snow/ski interface and the angle between skiis and the equipotential line), the lean angle of the subject during each phase of the turn can be calculated. Although another unknown angle would be necessary, namely, the one between the snow surface and the bottom of the ski, these information are enough to estimate the ground reaction forces that the lower limbs and trunk extensors need to contrast. In addition, body lean angle and centripetal force help to roughly assess the dynamic friction during turns, when assuming that there is no skidding. Coefficient of dynamic friction when skiing on a straight path was inferred by analysing the initial 30 m of the track, where subjects were instructed to let them be passively accelerated by gravity. Air drag was obtained from body speed and surface area and corrected according to literature estimates of skiers' drag coefficient. Needless to say that wind intensity and direction should be taken into account.

The results from this part of the experiment revealed that more than 50% of the total negative work needed for the descent is provided from air drag and snow/ski friction. That means that muscles 'have' to take care of at least 45% of it, which cor-responds to a lot of eccentric (lengthening) contractions. Also, the inspection of the total net mechanical energy of the body, which is in general monotonically decreas-ing, showed occasional increases (positive work) suggesting some positive work that could have been provided by a concentric muscle action, a release of elastic energy (see above) or a combination of the two effects in what is referred to as 'power ampli-fication' done by muscle-tendon interaction [5], a phenomenon allowing to obtain +40% more mechanical power than what is available from muscle alone. The final effect, namely, an increase of skier's speed beyond the mere exchange with body PE, deserves further attention, and its relevance will be likely assessed when technology will provide even more accurate 3D tracking of body motion.

As mentioned, though, that partitioning between 'passive' and 'active' negative work refers to giant slalom-like descents, it could be different for slalom, super-G and downhill races.

The quoted predictions, which rely just on nonbiological data, can be checked by analysing the signals from EMG electrodes and electrogoniometers. Time courses of joint angles detect flexion or extension, in the different phases of the descent, and reveal whether the relevant muscles are shortening or lengthening and at which speed they occur. EMG signals, being previously calibrated according to maximum voluntary isometric contractions (MVC) at different joint angles, allow to estimate the developed muscle force. Then, force development for muscle groups devoted to specific functions (hip, knee and ankle flexion or extension) can be analysed together with the collected video footage to reveal eccentric, isometric or eccentric actions in the different phases of skiing straight and during turns. Such a post-processing, whose complexity is addressable by using cross correlation algorithms from statistics, is currently ongoing and could potentially confirm the work partitioning suggested by kinematics.

Another important and peculiar biomechanical occurrence in Alpine ski is landing after a jump, which is spectacular particularly in downhill races. Again, it is a matter of energy dissipation, but there is no doubt here that eccentric muscle contraction is involved. The vertical downward speed builds up during the flight due to gravity, and high values of vertical momentum ($= mv_{vert}$) need to be suddenly lowered by joint extensor muscles at landing, which implies a substantial and accurately controlled force production during lengthening (negative work). Depending on the track configuration after landing, the skier faces two alternatives: (1) a fast reduction of vertical momentum to re-establish the correct posture as soon as possible or (2) a more progressive damping action, with much lower peaks of vertical ground reaction force. As high and sudden impacts during landing are associated with increased friction at the ski/snow interface, it is apparent that, to limit the unavoidable deceleration, the first option should be chosen only when racing posture is crucial to control the descent trajectory immediately after touchdown. The biomechanics of drop landing applied to Alpine ski indicates as a keyword the 'negative power', which is the ratio between negative work and damping duration [6]. It is very important, then, for athletes to be able to provide a very high negative power but also to modulate its delivery in a gradually controlled landing [7]. On this subject, the scientific literature is still quite scanty and further investigations are needed.

1.4   Conclusion and Future Perspectives

Alpine ski is a complex motor activity, very demanding both in terms of muscle performance and of neuromuscular control. The described approach for biomechanical research relies on comprehensive experiments where the time course of spatial coordinates and of biological signals (EMG and joint angles) from muscles needs to be sampled at a very high resolution and analysed synchronously with the video data. Despite that parts of the proposed research protocol have already been investigated (e.g. mechanical energy balance, [8, 9]; body kinetics, [10]; muscle control type, [11]), we are far from having a complete, representative description of how our musculoskeletal machine works in slalom, giant slalom, super-G and downhill skiing.

From all the illustrated information, it emerges that Alpine ski is dominated, ranked from the most important, by eccentric activity, followed by isometric and a potential small amount of concentric contraction (with or without the 'power amplification' effect of acting in combination with tendon recoil). We are in urgent need of a more deterministic science of snow/ski interaction, while the over-redundant constellation of geopositioning satellites, together with the modern technology of digital barometers, is expected to allow soon a very accurate and resoluted measurement of the skier trajectory along tracks.

This chapter deliberately disregarded many other biomechanical issues of Alpine skiing, particularly in relation to the upper portion of the body. It is the writer's opinion that a clear understanding of the 'engine' work is crucial to design training protocols and regimes that could enhance performance on the one hand and reduce injury chances during leisure and competitive skiing on the other hand.

References

1. Formenti F, Ardigó LP, Minetti AE (2005) Human locomotion on snow: determinants of economy and speed of skiing across the ages. Proc R Soc B 272(1572):1561–1569
2. Cerretelli P, Veicsteinas A, Fumagalli M, Dell'Orto L (1976) Energetics of isometric exercise in man. J Appl Physiol 41(2):136–141
3. Berg EB, Eiken O, Tesch PA (1995) Involvement of eccentric muscle actions in giant slalom racing. Med Sci Sports Exerc 27(12):1666–1670
4. Minetti AE (2017) Keynote Lecture. Concentric, isometric and eccentric contractions: which dominates alpine skiing? In: Müller E et al (eds) VIIth International Congress on Science and Skiing VII (ICSS), St. Cristoph, Austria, December, 2016. Meyer and Meyer Verlag, Aachen
5. Galantis A, Woledge RC (2003) The theoretical limits to the power output of a muscle-tendon complex with inertial and gravitational loads. Proc R Soc Biol Sci 270(1523):1493–1498
6. Minetti AE, Ardigò LP, Susta D, Cotelli F (1998) Using leg muscles as shock absorbers: theoretical predictions and experimental results of human drop landing. Ergonomics 41(12):1771–1791
7. Minetti AE, Susta D (2012) The maximum negative power and motor control during simulated hard and soft landing in alpine skiers. In: Müller E et al (eds) Vth International Congress on Science and Skiing, St Christoph, 2010. Science and Skiing V. Meyer and Meyer Verlag, Aachen, pp 291–297
8. Supej M, Kugovnik O, Nemec B (2012) Energy principle used for estimating the quality of a racing ski turn. In: Müller E et al (eds) Vth International Congress on Science and Skiing, St Christoph, 2010. Science and Skiing, V. Meyer and Meyer Verlag, Aachen, pp 228–237
9. Meyer F, Borrani F (2012) 3D model reconstruction and analysis of athletes performing giant slalom. In: Müller E et al (eds) Vth International Congress on Science and Skiing, St Christoph, 2010. Science and Skiing, V. Meyer and Meyer Verlag, Aachen, pp 272–281
10. Reid RC, Gilgien M, Kipp RW, Smith G (2012) Force and energy characteristic in competitive slalom. In: Müller E et al (eds) Vth International Congress on Science and Skiing, St Christoph, 2010. Science and Skiing, V. Meyer and Meyer Verlag, Aachen, pp 373–384
11. Kröll J, Spörri J, Fasel B, Müller E, Schwameder H (2014) Type of muscle control in elite Alpine skiing – is it still the same than in 1995? In: Müller E et al (eds) VIth International Congress on Science and Skiing, St Christoph, 2012. Science and Skiing, VI, pp 56–64

Chapter 2
Physiology of Alpine Skiing

Simone Porcelli and Marco Zancanaro

Abstract In alpine skiing, performance is determined by technical skills, and technical ability appears the greatest influencing factor. However, the ability to continually exhibit technical competence through each race and the long competitive season requires high physiological capabilities. The extreme environment characterized by cold and altitude makes ski racing more challenging under a physiological prospective. Thus, knowledge of the muscular forces and energy system usage in ski racing is important for future performance enhancement, injury prevention, talent identification, and training prescription.

2.1 Introduction

Alpine skiing is part of Winter Olympics since 1936 and consists of four traditional events, each differentiated by gate placement, turning radius, speed, and course length. All events require the skier to accelerate as quickly as possible from the starting gate to full speed before maintaining proper form and technique up to the end of the race. A downhill race (DH) may last as long as 2–3 min and a super giant slalom (SGS) race, which involves more turns but a shorter course, usually lasts 2 min. Giant slalom (GS) and slalom (SL) are slower and more technical events, with skiers only reaching 30–60 km/h. They are comprised of close together turns or gates, and each competitor makes two runs per day on the same slope, changing the position of the gates in the second run. GS typically lasts 60–90 s, while SL lasts 45–60 s [1, 2].

The physiological characteristics of skiers and requirements for the various events have been extensively described [3]. Elite alpine skiers are characterized by

S. Porcelli, MD, PhD
Institute of Molecular Bioimaging and Physiology, National Research Council,
LITA Building, Via Fratelli Cervi 93, 20090 Segrate, Milan, Italy
e-mail: simone.porcelli@ibfm.cnr.it

M. Zancanaro, MD
Winter Sports Italian Federation, Milan, Italy

superior dynamic balance ability, high leg strength, and high anaerobic and aerobic capacities [3]. Notably, these characteristics have changed across the years according to the shift in training and the demands of competition [4, 5]. Moreover, the introduction of new technologies has allowed and even encouraged greater skier physicality. For example, the carving ski has created a sharper, reduced radius turn, indirectly requiring greater muscle strength to cope with higher forces on lower limbs joints [6]. Today skiers' off-season and preseason training typically includes endurance and resistance training, inducing improvements in aerobic capacity, strength, and power [7]. During the competitive season, endurance and weight trainings are reduced, and on-snow time comprises 60–70% of total training. Accordingly, seasonal changes in the athletes' physical capacities can occur [8].

Data of Italian elite skiers collected in preseason and midseason periods are shown in Table 2.1. An increase in VO_2 max and maximal work can be observed, confirming the effects of different training sessions during competitive season. In literature a decreased isokinetic leg strength in postseason, compared with preseason, has been observed in international skiers in accordance with the reduction in specific endurance training [9]. In the same study, a decrease in VO_2 max was reported as concerning the reduction in specific endurance training during the competitive season.

2.2   Energy Supply During Skiing

The real contribution of aerobic and anaerobic metabolism during Alpine skiing is not known, and results of several studies are controversial. Technical events appear to rely more on anaerobic power, whereas the longer speed events incorporate greater contributions from aerobic metabolism [10]. Early investigations reported values of 80–90% VO_2 max for elite skiers [11]. Saibene et al. [12] calculated an aerobic demand of 120% VO_2 max during GS skiing. Veicsteinas et al. [13] found that the VO_2 of elite skiers was around 200% and 160% VO_2 max in SL and GS, respectively.

Table 2.2 reports the results of Veicsteinas et al. [13] and Saibene et al. [12]. Both studies used blood lactate measures to calculate total aerobic energy contribution, relying on the assumption that 1 mmol/L^{-1} blood lactate relates to 3.15 ml O_2/kg. The results show a 65% contribution from the anaerobic system in ski racing, suggesting the importance of muscle force and neuromuscular coordination in this sport [12, 13]. It should be noted that much of the skiing literature dates back to a period between the 1970s and 1990s. These studies reflect the demands of the sport as it was more than 20 years ago, before the influx of carving skis and specific training regimes [14]. Thus, the results must be reviewed critically as some of the investigative methods and technology used are now outdated.

There is no consensus about the importance of aerobic metabolism for ski racing [15]. Some authors state that maximal aerobic power is unlikely determinant for success

Table 2.1 Main physiological parameters obtained in skiers of the Italian national team during 2015/2016 and 2016/2017 seasons

		CMJ (cm)	W_{peak} (w)	VO_{2peak} (L·min⁻¹)	VO_{2peak} (mL·kg⁻¹·min⁻¹)	HR_{peak} (b·min⁻¹)	GET (L·min⁻¹)	GET (%VO_{2peak})
Pre-season	Women	39.2 ± 4.2	277 ± 29.0	2.949 ± 0.287	43.8 ± 3.0	194 ± 6	2.491 ± 0.233	84.6 ± 4.8
	Men	53.8 ± 5.6	419 ± 41.3	4.505 ± 0.409	52.6 ± 5.1	191 ± 10	3.838 ± 0.365	85.3 ± 5.1
Mid-season	Women	41.8 ± 4.8	286 ± 26.5	2.993 ± 0.339	44.3 ± 3.6	195 ± 6	2.470 ± 0.230	82.8 ± 5.1
	Men	54.5 ± 6.5	429 ± 43.7	4.825 ± 0.427	55.1 ± 5.4	193 ± 8	3.807 ± 0.365	84.7 ± 5.0

Table 2.2 Relative energy contribution to a single run on a ski race course

Author	Aerobic (%)	Lactic (%)	Phosphate (%)
Saibene et al. [11]	46.4	25.4	28.3
Veicsteinas et al. [12]	30–35	~40	25–30

Lactic contribution is estimated by calculating O_2 equivalent of lactic acid

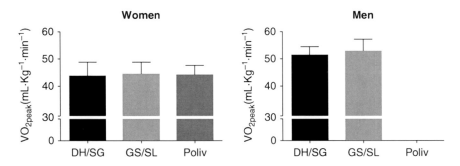

Fig. 2.1 VO_2 max of skiers of the Italian national team recorded during the season 2016/2017

in competitive alpine skiing, and it does not discriminate competitors of varying ability categories [1, 16]. On the other side, more recent studies have shown that aerobic power is strongly correlated with international skiing success [6]. Moreover, it should be noted that the utilization of the aerobic system during ski racing is complicated by physiological and environmental factors. For example, during skiing numerous isometric contractions required to generate muscle force induce sustained vascular occlusion [11, 17]. The resultant metabolic processes include muscle ischemia and hypoxia and altered ion concentration and substrate availability [18]. Therefore, muscle ischemia and a greater reliance on anaerobic metabolism occur, and glycogen utilization increases by up to 50% of pre-exercise levels [2]. Similarly, low temperature and hypoxic hypobaric environments result in reduced alveolar and arterial oxygen pressure, subsequently increasing glycolytic rates and reducing glycogen stores [18–22]. Indeed, Gladden and Welch [23] reported a 15% increase in anaerobic lactate system contribution to exercise during cycling at 120% VO_2 max at 2000 m above sea level. Accordingly, physiological parameters related to aerobic metabolism of alpine ski racers vary across different studies. For example, Saibene et al. [12] and Brown and Wilkinson [24] identified VO_2 max of 58.9 ± 2.17 mL kg^{-1} min^{-1} and 63.1 ± 1.3 mL kg^{-1} min^{-1}, respectively. Andersen and Montgomery [3] reported much higher values (67 mL kg^{-1} min^{-1}), while Veicsteinas et al. [13] reported lower values (52 mL kg^{-1} min^{-1}). Recent data on the world champion Austrian team identify values of 59.5 ± 4.7 mL kg^{-1} min^{-1} and 58.7 ± 3.2 mL kg^{-1} min^{-1} for the 1999 and 2000 seasons, respectively [6]. Figure 2.1 shows the VO_2 max of skiers of the Italian national team recorded during the season 2016/2017. Each column represents data obtained from athletes of different disciplines.

Usually, aerobic metabolism is tested in the laboratory by incremental running exercises on a treadmill. However, many skiers lack running technique and may be limited by low back pain during this kind of exercise [22, 24]. As a consequence, cycling exercises rather than treadmill running are preferred in ski racers and in these last year's incremental cycle step tests to determine onset of blood lactate accumulation and VO_2 max have been used to assess skiers [6, 14, 25].

As for anaerobic metabolism, some studies show that anaerobic power tests, especially when adjusted for body mass, are significantly correlated with ski performance. White [1] reported that vertical jump was the best indicator of skier performance, while Haymes and Dickinson [26] found vertical jump to correlate well with FIS points. Today, anaerobic metabolism is usually evaluated by Wingate test. While the 30s Wingate appears to be the most commonly used test, the 60s and 90s tests have become more popular and may be more relevant to the time scales and energy systems involved in ski racing. Bacharach and Duvillard [15] SL skiers have greater maximal power outputs but are unable to sustain these for long periods, while conversely DH racers were able to sustain higher average power outputs for longer but showed lower maximal powers. Alternatively, blood lactate can be easily used as an indicator of anaerobic contribution to energy supply and metabolic acidosis.

2.3   Muscular Strength

Skiing is often defined as an "explosive" sport, according to the accelerative forces resulting from fast downhill skiing, combined with successive sharp forceful slalom turns [27]. However, some studies showed slower angular knee velocities in ski racing compared to running and demonstrated very high leg strength only when tested at slow movement velocities (i.e., 30°/s) [1, 28]. Moreover, it is well known that eccentric actions are the prevalent muscle contractive force during ski racing [28]. Such a dominance of eccentric load has not been reported in other sports, and is thought to result from continuous downward displacement, negating the need for the forceful concentric actions typical of running and jumping [17, 28]. Such findings suggest that strength training for skiing should include a predominance of eccentric activity [27, 28].

From a physiological prospective, it has been suggested that high strength level may allow the athlete to work at a reduced percentage of their maximum voluntary contraction, thereby reducing the metabolic consequences of sustained high-intensity activity and the risk of injuries [2, 17, 29]. Indeed, insufficient strength may limit a skiers' ability to withstand the high forces and eccentric loads of ski racing. This may results in significant increases in valgus subluxation forces within the knee joint and subsequent joint dislocations and/or ligaments rupture. From this prospective, particular attention is aimed to the ratio of hamstring to quadriceps strength, which is used to identify predisposition to such injury. Neumayr et al. [6] found hamstring/quadriceps ratios of 0.57–0.60 among a group of world champion skiers, indicating good controlling hamstring strength relative to power producing quadriceps activity.

It is important to note that poor hamstring/quadriceps ratio strength in lower level athletes has been reported, particularly due to weak hamstrings. Thus, trainers should be aware of hamstring importance among younger ski racers.

Isokinetic dynamometry, utilizing leg extension (and sometimes leg flexion), has become the standard laboratory tool for assessing leg strength in skiers as it is able to accurately identify concentric, isometric, and eccentric torque at various joint velocities. Explosive power measures have also universally utilized, and they involve a vertical jump, repeated vertical jumps, or double- and single-leg bounding [1, 30, 31].

2.4   Future Prospectives

Much of the current skiing literature describes the energy demands of a single ski run, and little attention has been paid to the physiological requirements of multiple day race training. Quantification of energy consumption, muscle damage, and nutritional requirements of several days of high-intensity race training should be pursued. Moreover, ski research is often descriptive, and it focuses on short term. To clearly understand ski racing and how performance may be altered by physical conditioning, we need longitudinal studies to be performed. Tracking of athletes, from their initiation to top-level racing, and their physiological progression with maturity, matched with that of skill and performance success, may highlight what type of athlete can be a successful skier. Such information may be helpful for talent identification and training periodization [15].

Considering the conflicting reports of aerobic and anaerobic requirements in ski racing, more specific physiological measurements of world class skiers, with special reference to tissue oxidization, fiber type, mitochondrial density, and enzymatic differences, are also necessary. In particular, further investigation into fiber type distribution and metabolism, with respect to the capacity of the athlete to cope with cold, altitude, high force, and ischemic conditions, is necessary.

Finally, innovative technology such as EMG, video, and GPS should be utilized more to, for example, identify specific athlete requirements based upon course type (technical or speed) and terrain (steepness and snow/ice condition) [1].

2.5   Conclusions

Ski racing is a multifaceted sport, and no singular feature can be used to predict success in alpine skiing. Technical skills are fundamental, and the training on the snow should cover most of the training time of the athletes. Nevertheless, a thorough understanding of the physiological demands of ski racing must be pursued in order to ensure precise, quality training without wasted time or effort. Skiers train and compete in extreme environments of cold, altitude, and sustained high-force muscle contractions. These conditions make investigation difficult and the physiological demands of ski racing hard to accurately quantify. Thus, further research should aim to understand the specific physiological costs of ski racing and the usefulness of aerobic versus anaerobic training methodologies, given advances in both ski technique and technology. Moreover, it is essential to establish accurate profiles of current, world's leading athletes, to appropriately structure training and periodization programs. During periods of intense competition, where technical and physical training becomes limited, through lack of training facilities, time, or finance, it is important that what little training is performed is both effective and relevant.

References

1. White AT, Johnson SC (1993) Physiological aspects and injury in elite alpine skiers. Sports Med 15(3):170–178
2. Szmedra L, Im J, Nioka S, Chance B, Rundell W (2001) Hemoglobin/myoglobin oxygen desaturation during alpine skiing. Med Sci Sport Exer 33(2):232–236
3. Andersen RE, Montgomery DL (1988) Physiology of alpine skiing. Sports Med 6:210–221
4. Müller E, Benko U, Raschner C, Schwameder H (1998) Specific fitness training and testing in competitive sports. Med Science in Sport Exer 32(1):216–220
5. Stōlen T, Chamari K, Castagna C, Wisolff U (2005) Physiology of soccer: an update. Sports Med 35(6):510–536
6. Neumayr G, Hoertnagl H, Pfister R, Koller A, Eibl G, Raas E (2003) Physical and physiological factors associated with success in professional alpine skiing. Int J Sports Med 34:571–575
7. Steadman RJ, Swanson KR, Atkins JW, Hangerman GR (1987) Training for alpine skiing. Clin Orthop Relat Res 216:34–38
8. Bosco C, Cotelli F, Bonomi R, Mogononi P, Roi GS (1994) Seasonal fluctuations of selected physiological characteristics of elite alpine skier. Eur J Appl Physiol 69:71–74
9. Koutedakis Y, Boreham C, Kabitsis C, Sharp NCC (1992) Seasonal deterioration of selected physiological variables in elite male skiers. Int J Sport Med 13:548–551
10. Duvillard SP (1995) Introduction: the interdisciplinary approach to the science of alpine skiing. Med Sci Sport Exer 27(3):303–304
11. Tesch P, Larsson L, Eriksson A, Karlsson J (1978) Muscle glycogen depletion and lactate concentration during downhill skiing. Med Sci Sports 10(2):85–90
12. Saibene F, Cortili G, Gavazzi P, Magistri P (1985) Energy sources in alpine skiing (giant slalom). Eur J Appl Physiol 55:312–316
13. Veicsteinas A, Ferretti G, Margonato V, Rosa G, Tagliabue D (1984) Energy cost of and energy sources for alpine skiing in top athletes. J Appl Physiol 56:1187–1190
14. Karlsonn J (2005) Alpine skiing physiology: retro and prospectus. In: Muller E, Bacharach D, Klika R, Lindinger S, Schwameder H (eds) Science and skiing II. Meyer & Meyer Sport (UK) Ltd, Oxford, pp 24–38
15. Bacharach DW, Duvillard SP (1995) Intermediate and long-term anaerobic performance of elite alpine skiers. Med Sci Sport Exer 27(3):305–309
16. Tesch PA (1995) Aspects on muscle properties and use in competitive alpine skiing. Med Sci Sport Exercise 27(3):310–314
17. Foster C, Rundell KW, Snyder AC, Stray-Gundersen J, Kemkers G, Thometz N, Broker J, Knapp E (1999) Evidence for restricted muscle blood flow during speed skating. Med Sci Sports Exerc 31(10):1433–1440

18. Seifert JG, Kipp RW, Amann M, Gazal O (2005) Muscle damage, fluid ingestion and energy supplementation during recreational alpine skiing. Int J Sport Nutr Exerc Metab 15:528–536
19. Kuno S-Y, Inaki M, Tanaka K, Itai Y, Asano K (1994) Muscle energetics in short-term training during hypoxia in elite combination skiers. Eur J Appl Physiol 69:301–304
20. Haman F, Peronnet F, Kenny GP, Massicotte D, Lavoie C, Scott C, Weber JM (2002) Effects of cold exposure on fuel utilization in humans: plasma glucose, muscle glycogen, and lipids. J Appl Physiol 93:77–84
21. Roberts D (2005) Induction of endogenous erythropoietin: hypoxic exercise or natremic stimulus? In: Muller E, Bacharach D, Klika R, Lindinger S, Schwameder H (eds) Science and skiing II. Meyer & Meyer Sport (UK) Ltd, Oxford, pp 39–55
22. Svensson MD (2005) Testing soccer players. J Sports Sci 23(6):610–618
23. Gladden LB, Welch HG (1978) Efficiency of anaerobic work. J Appl Physiol Respir Environ Exerc Physiol 44(4):564–570
24. Brown SL, Wilkinson JG (1983) Characteristics of national, divisional and club male alpine ski racers. Med Sci Sport Exer 15(6):491–495
25. Noe F, Paullard T (2005) Is postural control affected by expertise in alpine skiing. Br J Sports Med 39:835–837
26. Haymes EM, Dickinson AL (1980) Characteristics of elite male and female ski racers. Med Sci Sport Exer 12(3):153–158
27. Berg HE, Eiken O, Tesch PA (1995) Involvement of eccentric muscle actions in giant slalom racing. Med Sci Sport Exer 27(12):1666–1670
28. Berg HE, Eiken O (1999) Muscle control in elite alpine skiing. Med Sci Sports Exerc 31(7):1065–1067
29. Rundell CF (1996) Compromised oxygen uptake in speed skaters during treadmill in-line skating. Med Sci Sports Exerc 28(1):120–127
30. Andersen RE, Montgomery DL, Turcotte RA (1990) An on-site test battery to evaluate giant slalom skiing performance. J Sports Med Phys Fitness 30(3):276–282
31. White AT, Johnson SC (1991) Physiological comparison of international, national and regional alpine skiers. Int J Sports Med 12:374–378

Chapter 3
Training and Testing for Elite Skiers

Roberto Manzoni and Andrea Viano

Abstract Alpine skiing is a sport spread all over the world. Several elements contribute to athletic performance: technical, tactical, psychological and physical. In this chapter we will analyse different training methods applied to elite alpine skiers and describe classical functional tests utilised to monitoring performance changes.

3.1 Background

Over the years both the training methods and the evaluation tests of alpine ski athletes have changed. We have moved from the concept of targeted training for the technical gesture to individualised training for each individual athlete.

3.2 Competitive Alpine Skiing

At the international level, this discipline is governed by the International Ski Federation (FIS). The discipline "alpine skiing" includes several competitive disciplines: downhill (DH) (vertical drop 800–1100 m, 1 run), slalom (SL) (vertical drop 180–220 m, no. of direction changes 30–35% of vertical drop, 2 runs), giant slalom (GS) (vertical drop 250–450 m, no. of direction changes 11–15% of vertical drop, 2 runs), super-G (SG) (vertical drop 400–650 m, no. of direction changes at least 7% of vertical drop, 1 run) and combined [alpine and classical (DH-SG and SL 1 run, DH and SL 1 run)].

Competitive events are divided by gender and by age categories, and they range from local junior competitions to national and absolute continental cups (the first World Cup skiing competition was held in 1967) to world cups (seasonal circuit and

R. Manzoni (✉) • A. Viano
National Alpine Ski Team, Italian Winter Sport Federation, Milan, Italy
e-mail: roberto.manzoni2014@gmail.com

© Springer International Publishing AG 2018   17
H. Schoenhuber et al. (eds.), *Alpine Skiing Injuries*, Sports and Traumatology,
https://doi.org/10.1007/978-3-319-61355-0_3

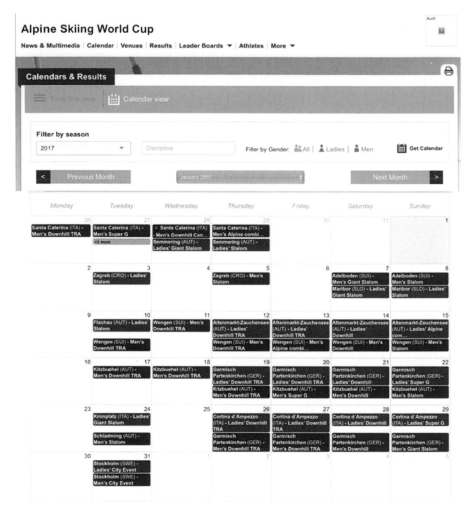

Fig. 3.1 Calendar for the women's and men's World Cup, January 2017. Note the density of events and consider the travelling required to reach the competition sites

biennial event) and Olympic Games (winter games, held in Chamonix every 4 years since 1924).

In 2013/2014, from October to March, the FIS organised 69 World Cup competitions for men and women at 28 sites in 12 different countries (Fig. 3.1).

3.3   Competitive Alpine Skiing: Classification

Some authors consider alpine skiing to be a discipline requiring "...dexterity and muscle strength, mixed aerobic-anaerobic metabolic activity with predominance of the anaerobic (alactic and lactic) over the aerobic component" [1].

Others classify the four specialties (SL, GS, SG, DH) of alpine skiing "… among the sports with immediate adaptation of posture and/or skis to the environment" [2].

Hébert-Losier et al. [3] stated that to efficiently use the potential energy possessed at the start, during the descent the athlete must minimise the friction resulting both from ski-snow contact and from aerodynamic drag. Therefore choosing the most appropriate trajectory for the course means maintaining a high velocity of descent. For this to be possible, the athlete must practise both in training and in competition his or her individual techniques and tactics (e.g. consistent with his or her individual traits). The authors also note that the best run times are almost invariably recorded for good average velocities developed across all sections of the course rather than for velocity peaks in short sections (resulting from differences in snow, slope, course, etc.). This emphasises that the factor that most limits performance lies in the technical-tactical components, in the ongoing quest for optimal biomechanical parameters and in the extremely high muscular load intensity.

3.4   Competitive Alpine Skiing: The Skiers

On its official website (www.fis-ski.com), the FIS records and reports the quantitative data on current alpine ski racers. To date, it counts no less than 15,972 members in 81 countries (Figs. 3.2 and 3.3).

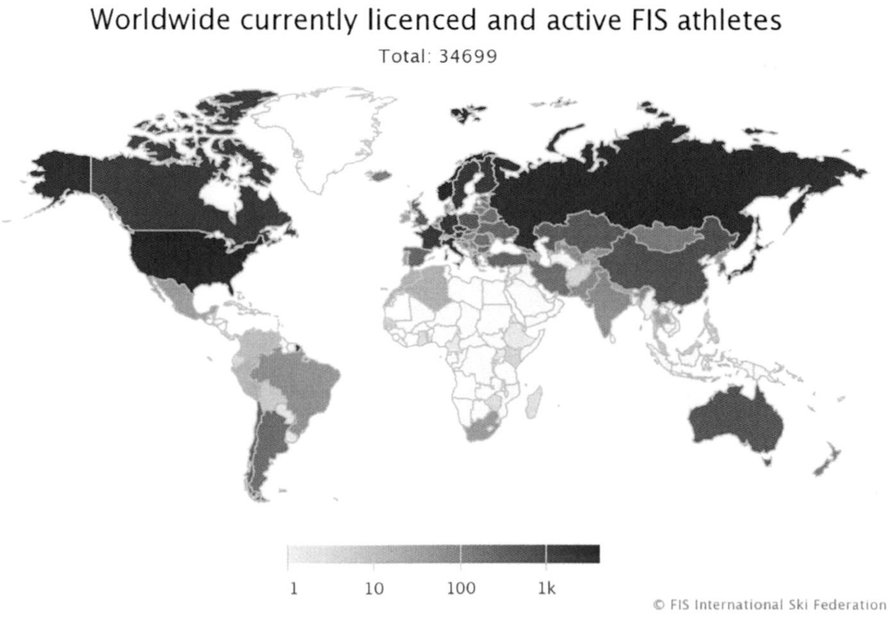

Worldwide currently licenced and active FIS athletes
Total: 34699

1   10   100   1k

© FIS International Ski Federation

Fig. 3.2 Number of FIS athletes worldwide as of December 2016

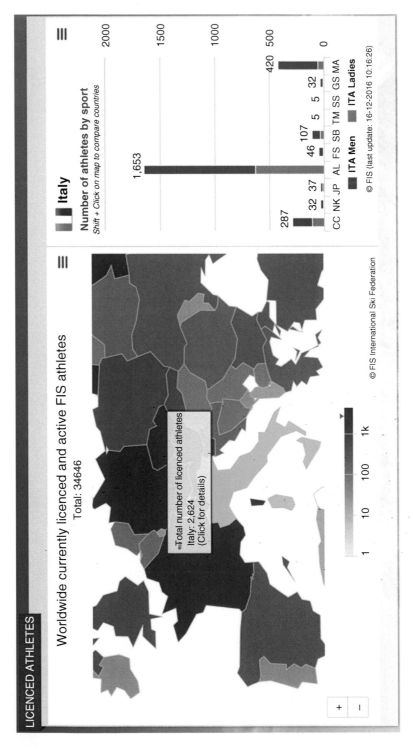

Fig. 3.3 Number of FIS athletes in Italy and in particular in alpine skiing (AL)

3.5   Competitive Alpine Skiing: The Performance Model

A performance model refers to the objective definition of a number of biological factors that characterise or limit performance. Clearly these measured data must be able to guide and assess the athlete's training.

The recognised components of performance are technical (predominant), tactical, psychological and physical. The physical factors are essentially assessed by determining the muscle strength (eccentric and concentric) used in curves (especially after the advent of carving skis) and the manner in which the energy systems produce energy (VO_2 max and glycolysis) and recover from fatigue (blood and neuromuscular lactate).

Many researchers have attempted this difficult task.

Alpine skiing is a complex sport in which competition performance is the result of both physical and technical factors. The races are characterised by high-intensity physical actions lasting 60–120 s on average, in which a series of very strong, predominantly eccentric and isometric contractions occur in rapid succession [4].

For these reasons, in alpine skiing aerobic capacity, strength, muscle power and fatigue tolerance are all crucial physical factors for elite athletes [5, 6].

Gilgien [7] and Muller [8] reported force values exceeding 2000 N, as recorded by GPS, accelerometers and mathematical models.

Reid and Gigien (2012) found forces equal to 3–4 G in SL.

Hintermeister [9] recorded the EMG signal of lower limb and trunk muscles via telemetry on seven GS and SL elite skiers. During the curve the values detected were between 58 and 125% of MVC (maximum voluntary contraction). Similar values were recorded both during SL and GS, with significant qualitative differences in activation of the tibialis anterior during SL and external oblique during GS.

Berg [10] performed EMG on 16 athletes of the Swedish national team finding greater activation in the late phases of eccentric contraction, with values at times higher than 100% of MVC.

In his 2010 paper, "Limitations to performance during alpine skiing", Ferguson summarises the features of the sport as follows:

1. It is a high-intensity exercise.
2. It has a duration ranging from 90 to 120 s.
3. It is characterised by repeated phases of high-force isometric and eccentric contractions.
4. This leads to a restriction of blood flow with consequent reduction in oxygen supply.
5. It produces both central (systems) and peripheral (neuromuscular) fatigue.
6. It is capable of impairing motor control (technique).

In their well-known (and much discussed) paper "Physical and physiological factors associated with success in professional alpine skiing", Neumayr et al. [6] investigated the metabolic and muscular features of the Austrian World Cup ski team over the years 1997–2000. In addition to the usual anthropometric data, the study focused on the prevalent crucial factors of performance, i.e. it measured the indexes of aerobic power and strength of the lower limbs. The values measured were truly remarkable, as regards both the male and female Austrian World Cup ski teams of the time.

The researcher Bjørnar Haaland, in his 2015 master's thesis in Sports Physiotherapy at the Department of Sports Medicine of the Norwegian School of Sport Sciences [11] "Injury rate and injury patterns in FIS World Cup Alpine Skiing: have the new ski regulations made an impact?", in the section entitled "Physical characteristics of alpine skiers", states: "Alpine ski racing demands aerobic and anaerobic power, muscular strength and a set of various complex motoric skills, such as coordination, balance, agility and adeptness. The physical characteristics vary between disciplines. Ski racers competing in the technical events have been found to weigh less on average than the racers in speed events. In general, alpine ski racers have very high leg strength compared with other athletes".

In conclusion, it is clear that the actual contribution to performance of the various energy systems remains a difficult area to investigate because of the effect of individual and situational parameters and the technical movements made throughout the competition.

All of the studies acknowledge that biomechanics alone, as investigated on the individual athlete, for a single curve, on a specific slope and with unique snow conditions, has limited utility in helping to understand the phenomenon. All authors emphasise the need for studies taking into account the complexity of the issue, including differences among athletes, environmental factors and, above all, technical factors.

3.6   Competitive Alpine Skiing: Brief History of Sports Training

Sports training has a fairly recent history. It was the early twentieth century when the athletes participating in the first modern Olympic Games found a way to promote and represent their countries in sport and even politically. Eastern European countries in particular invested in this field. Sports and sports training sciences were founded, and physicians, biomechanics specialists and psychologists started to investigate the phenomenon. The figure of the coach developed.

The first sports to be investigated were obviously the Olympic sports, especially track and field and gymnastics. Sports training became a rational science: studying the most effective and efficient technique, identifying athletes based on anatomical and biological criteria, spotting and supporting talents and building periodised performance all became habitual. Athletes enjoyed a privileged social status on the grounds that they were represented and expressed by an entire nation.

For decades, the culture of the former Soviet Union exerted its influence worldwide. Constructing preparatory drills, planning training loads, alternating training and recovery and looking after the athlete's health (doping excluded) became the cornerstones of training based on early quantitative criteria.

In winter sports and in particular in alpine skiing, this new trend arrived in Italy with some delay. It was only in the 1980s that track and field coaches were engaged as physical trainers. Initially these physical trainers were not sport specific although over the years, partly thanks to federal initiatives, they came to develop an increasing number of specific competencies.

More recently, as a result of major biological, psychological and social changes coupled with the findings of applied research, there has been a shift from an exclusively physical and quantitative approach to training to sensory-neurological-motor training methods based on recognition that, athletic level being equal, the role of technique is predominant. Training methods are increasingly grounded in scientific evidence of effectiveness. Given the epidemiology of injury in competitive alpine skiing, prevention and interprofessional team management of the training programme have become key concepts in addition to performance.

3.7 Competitive Alpine Skiing: Training Practice

To summarise, alpine skiing, in its different technical forms and four specialties, can be defined as an open-air sport practised at high altitude and at low environmental temperature. Competitions are timed circuits with a high coordination, technical and tactical component. Its peculiarities are related to high-speed sliding, capable of generating extremely high muscular and articular tensions. Competitions have a duration between 45″ and 1′30″ per run for GS and SL (to be repeated twice). For SG and DH, the length can exceed 2′.

The training programme of the Italian national teams is managed, according to a consolidated model, by an interprofessional team that includes technical coaches, a physical trainer, a physiotherapist, an equipment technician and a physician, in addition to the athletes (in varying numbers depending on the discipline and objectives).

The work is carried out as a team, but the programme is tailored to the individual athlete. The combination of technical skill, athletic capabilities, quality of equipment and psychological-physical health will inevitably lead to personalised choices.

The team's project will therefore start from the individual and his or her specific characteristics. A functional assessment is the first step in planning and programming competitive goals.

To better understand FISI's approach to the physical training of elite alpine skiers, below we briefly present the thematic areas developed by the national teams' trainers to document the guidelines adopted.

3.8   Competitive Alpine Skiing: Guidelines
for Physical Training

1. Functional-attitudinal assessment: this will be widely discussed in the next section.
2. Warm-up—post-activation potentiation—cool-down: this has become a very popular topic since a new line of research revealed the limited attention paid to this aspect in preparing the competition. More than just a thermal warm-up, it is an overall activation (the key seems to be hormonal and neuromuscular) to be carried out over the hours and minutes preceding the start. Even after the arrival, specific procedures can be used to improve recovery from fatigue.
3. Joint mobility—functional stability: the whole culture of muscular elasticity (stretching) is being reconsidered. The guiding principle considers muscle as a means to provide joint control and active stability.
4. Muscle strength: the lengthy classifications of muscle strength expressions have been replaced by the ability to dose muscle strength. As a contractile organ, a muscle is able to develop mechanical tensions. It is therefore the load the muscle is responding to that will determine the type of tension, through continuous feedback with the nervous system. Given the discipline's performance model (strength/velocity), strength training is aimed at the quality of the movement. The load to be moved (usually a barbell) will therefore be correlated with the ergonomics, speed and amplitude of the movement, parameters that have come to replace series and repetitions.
5. Core and peripheral resistance: the role of aerobic power in alpine skiing performance has long been debated, and there now appears to be some agreement in considering oxygen metabolism highly important in the overall economy of long training and competition season, though not directly fundamental for performance in the single competition.
6. Speed and rapidity: skiing is defined as the "fastest non-motorised sport on Earth" and "the sport with the highest risk of injury ever undertaken by man". These two aspects of the discipline call for special care for this motor skill closely related to the neuromuscular system.
7. Skill and learning: when the neuromuscular system (see above) is unable to support feedback-directed control, feedforward structures need to be harnessed, that is, acquired knowledge and experience allowing the athlete to predict what will happen along the course (during competitions or training). This refers to the "old" coordination skills that remind us that learning is a skill that needs to be persistently refined. Learning is enhanced every time the exercise is new, interesting, fun, consistent with the athlete's abilities and organised in a taxonomic manner.
8. Timed circuits: ability to synthesise. Neuromuscular and metabolic resources need to be combined with motor and tactical skills. In our experience, timed circuits prove to be the most sport-specific instrument. The "time" variable and the possibility of having various setups for the workout stations make them highly effective.
9. Core training: as an educational and preventive tool.

10. Training monitoring: this refers to the collection of data and information about:
    - External load (the content of training)
    - Internal load (the effects produced on the individual athlete)
    - Physical and psychological well-being
    - Enjoyment of the training sessions
    - Quality of sleep
    - Nutritional plan

    Monitoring an athlete's training load is important for establishing whether the programme is achieving the desired adaptation and for minimising the risk of overreaching, injury and illness. Training monitoring is necessary for short- and long-term programming.

    An individualised approach is necessary to guarantee that the internal load perceived by the athlete corresponds to the trainer's expectations. One of the commonly reported objectives of training monitoring is the prevention of injuries.

11. Transfer: given the environmental and seasonal specificity of winter sports, during certain periods of the year, the athletes will practise other sports. The choice of sport should take into account the athlete's preference without however neglecting the performance model.

12. Prevention: see the final sections of Chaps. 7 and 8.

3.9 Competitive Alpine Skiing: Functional Assessment of the Athlete

Motor testing should be (must be!) the means (and not the end!) for objectively determining an individual's (athlete's) skill and predisposition for a given sport. The performance model discussed above demands that we establish the best test (or test battery) for assessing the skill we intend to measure. Clearly, this should be done by using rigorous procedures and reliable instruments.

The motor test is used to quantify, plan and check the progress of training for the single athlete and to compare this progress with a sample of subjects of the same qualification level.

The motor test is the initial step in a sports project. It provides the basis for planning the content of a short-, middle- and long-term training programme.

What tests should be used for functional assessments in alpine skiing has long been debated. As early as the 1980s–1990s, a number of eminent Italian and international scientists and physiologists (such as Saibene, Veicsteinas, Mognoni, Berg and Eiken) studied this sport in the laboratory and by means of applied physiology field studies without, however, ever identifying a variable capable of correlating technical performance and laboratory data. Neither anthropometric characteristics nor oxygen metabolism, nor muscle strength (in all its forms), nor any motor skill (balance, rhythm, etc.) was indeed able to completely explain performance in this complex discipline.

Therefore the best way to interpret and tackle performance is probably to consider it a complex system to be dealt with as such, that is, by studying each of its components, working as an interprofessional team and heavily involving the athlete as the central character of this "film".

To assess the male and female athletes of the eight national alpine skiing teams, for the past three seasons the Italian Federation of Winter Sports has been relying on the collaboration of "MAPEI SPORT", a centre based in Olgiate Olona (Varese).

The test battery administered to the athletes is the result of deep, scientific speculations. The Federal Medical Committee and the physical trainers of the Competition Directorate have, together with the laboratory experts, devised a sequence of assessments aiming to provide the athletes' training teams with useful information.

The test battery undertaken by the athletes of the Italian national alpine skiing teams consists of an anthropometric assessment to determine body fat percentage, a functional movement screen (FMS), an incremental exercise test on a cycle ergometer to measure peak oxygen consumption (VO_{2peak}), a vertical jump test with countermovement on a force platform and a specific fatigue resistance test involving a simulation on a Mognoni eccentric press. The aims of the test battery are to assess the most important physical qualities for a skier and to monitor the changes produced by the summer training period. More in detail:

1. *Blood chemistry:* general health status.
2. *Anthropometric assessment:* measurement of height and body weight and estimation of body fat percentage using the skinfold test [12].
3. *Functional movement screen:* performance of seven specific "key" movements representing an individual's normal, non-pathological movement function. The test screens for possible limitations or asymmetries that an individual may exhibit in performing those movements.
4. *Incremental exercise test on a cycle ergometer:* pedalling on an exercise bicycle in the lab following a protocol involving 25 W increments per minute starting from an intensity of 100 W. The athlete is strongly encouraged to reach his or her maximal performance to allow measurement of VO_{2peak} and peak power output (PPO). Additionally, ventilatory anaerobic threshold (point of respiratory compensation) and heart rate are also evaluated.
5. *Vertical jump test:* performance of a series of vertical jumps with countermovement on a force platform (Kistler Quattro Jump). The main parameters tested are the height of the jump, peak force and peak power developed during the test.
6. *Simulation on a Mognoni eccentric press:* a unique test carried out on a specific motorised horizontal press devised by Prof. Piero Mognoni and developed by Mapei Sport. The athletes perform three series (20″, 60″ and 90″, respectively) of standardised eccentric-concentric contractions separated by a 3′ rest. The athlete's goal is to try and maintain the same force level during the contractions of the same series. The required force level is calculated based on the athlete's body weight and differs between men and women: 2.8 and 1.9 times the body weight,

respectively, for the eccentric and concentric contraction for men and 2.5 and 1.7 times the body for women. At the end of each series, electrical stimulation of the peripheral femoral nerve is used to determine the quadriceps's ability to generate force, and the athlete's vertical jump capabilities are measured. The Mognoni leg press simulation assesses the degree of lower limb fatigue, and therefore the athlete's ability to resist ski-specific fatigue.

3.9.1   Competitive Alpine Skiing: Functional Assessment and Reference Tables

Generated by data processing, these reference tables are used to study each single athlete (the different bars) in relation to a reference sample. The vertical dashed lines distinguish a low level, an intermediate level and an excellent level among the athletes.

Incremental maximal exercise test on a cycle ergometer to determine maximum oxygen consumption and power peak is shown in Fig. 3.4.

3.9.2   Competitive Alpine Skiing: Functional Assessment and Personal Reports

The results of the assessment are immediately processed and made available. A meeting of the athlete and training team with the laboratory expert allows evaluation of the current situation and planning of future interventions.

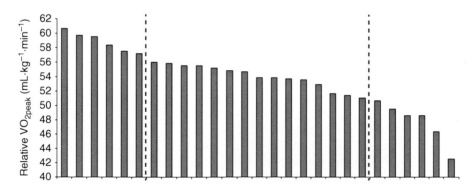

Fig. 3.4 Individual values of maximum oxygen consumption expressed in relative terms (VO_{2peak}, $mL·kg^{-1}·min^{-1}$) reached on the incremental exercise test on a cycle ergometer for the male athletes of the Italian national alpine skiing teams during the first functional assessment

3.10   Competitive Alpine Skiing: From Long-Term Athlete Development (LTAD) to Long-Term Skier Development (LTSD)

The concept of LTAD, or long-term development of the athlete, arises from awareness of the shortcomings of recent projects for talent identification and support projects undertaken by different countries and agencies and from the need to contextualise the issue of sports within modern society. It was discovered that athletes often do not follow organised training pathways but come from a multisport, fun and passionate juvenile experience and a late sport specialisation.

Scientific evidence has shown that LTAD has proven to be not only a mechanism capable of actively contrasting the sad phenomenon of athletes dropping out at an early age (due to boredom or frustration) but also the most powerful tool for preventing injuries and limiting the associated healthcare costs. It is predicted that such an organised system will develop potential talents and allow those not endowed with outstanding qualities to continue to do sports and keep fit.

The model is based on a number of principles:

1. Recognition of the biological-psychological characteristics of young developing athletes. Often biological age does not correspond to chronological age.
2. Active involvement and participation of families and institutions (public administration, school, sports clubs, etc.).
3. Subdivision of interventions into chronological pedagogical-educational phases (never rigid!).
4. Quality of trainers-educators must be very high.
5. Guidelines envisaging the development of "anthropological" motor patterns necessary for preparing a healthy young athlete/future champion capable of excellent performance.

Internationally, several LTAD models have been applied to the different sports. Among them, the Canadian model stands out which has been applied by both the winter and summer sports federations. Other countries that have embraced this approach are Great Britain for gymnastics and cycling, Australia for swimming and rugby and Germany and Belgium for soccer schools. As regards alpine skiing, in addition to Canada, the model has been adopted in the United States, Scandinavia and a number of European countries.

An ongoing project of the Italian Federation of Winter Sports is to create an LTAD model specific for alpine skiing, known as LTSD (long-term skier development) that takes into account the country's needs and its geographical, social, cultural, economic and institutional peculiarities.

The LTSD model aims to provide guidelines for both the technical and athletic-mental components, engaging different players such as parents, coaches, teachers, club managers and obviously the athletes themselves.

The various phases of LTSD lie along a developmental pathway that starts from "start of activity" to go on to "skier fundamentals", "learning to train" and "learning to compete" and finally "training to win". An equally important, closely related phase is "skiing for life".

References

1. Chicco Cotelli, Mario Cotelli (2008) Sci moderno. La storia degli ultimi 40 anni. La ricerca scientifica. Le quattro discipline. Mulatero Editore
2. Claudio Scotton (2003) Classificazione tecnica delle Discipline Sportive. Calzetti Mariucci Editore
3. Hébert-Losier K, Supej M, Holmberg HC (2014) Biomechanical factors influencing the performance of elite alpine ski racers. Sports Med 44:519–533
4. Ferguson RA (2010) Limitations to performance during alpine skiing. Exp Physiol 95(3):404–410
5. Tesch PA (1995) Aspects on muscle properties and use in competitive alpine skiing. Med Sci Sports Exerc 27(3):310–314
6. Neumayr G, Hoertnagl H, Pfister R, Koller A, Eibl G, Raas E (2003a) Physical and physiological factors associated with success in professional alpine skiing. Int J Sports Med 24:571–575
7. Gilgien M, Spörri J, Chardonnens J, Kröll J, Müller E (2013) Determination of external forces in alpine skiing using a differential global navigation satellite system. Sensors 13(8):9821–9835
8. Müller E, Schwameder H (2003) Biomechanical aspects of new techniques in alpine skiing and ski-jumping. J Sport Sci 21:679–692. Published online: 13 Jun 2008
9. Hintermeister RA, O'Connor DD, Dillman CJ, Suplizio CL, Lange GW, Steadman JR (1995) Muscle activity in slalom and giant slalom skiing. Med Sci Sports Exerc 27(3):315–322
10. Berg HE, Eiken O (1999) Muscle control in elite alpine skiing. Med Sci Sport Exer 31(7):1065–1067
11. Haaland B (2015) Injury rate and injury patterns in FIS World Cup Alpine Skiing: have the new ski regulations made an impact? Master thesis in Sports Physiotherapy, Department of Sports Medicine, Norwegian School of Sport Sciences
12. Jackson AS, Pollock ML (1978) Generalized equations for predicting body density of men. Br J Nutr 40:497

Further Reading

Federolf P, Reid R, Gilgien M, Haugen P, Smith G (2014) The application of principal component analysis to quantify technique in sports. Scand J Med Sci Sports 24:491–499

Turnbull JR, Kilding AE, Keogh WL (2009) Physiology of alpine skiing. Scand J Med Sci Sports 19(2):146–155

Kümmel J, Kramer A, Giboin LS, Gruber M (2016) Specificity of balance training in healthy individuals: a systematic review and meta-analysis. Sports Med 46(9):1261–1271

Supej M, Senner V, Petrone N, Holmberg HC (2017) Reducing the risks for traumatic and overuse injury among competitive alpine skiers. Br J Sports Med 51(1):1–2

Huxel Bliven KC, Anderson BE (2013) Core stability training for injury prevention. Sports Health 5(6):514–522

Hoppeler H (2016) Moderate load eccentric exercise: a distinct novel training modality. Front Physiol 7:483

Zebis MK, Bencke J, Andersen LL et al (2011) Acute fatigue impairs neuromuscular activity of anterior cruciate ligament-agonist muscles in female team handball players. Scand J Med Sci Sports 21(6):833–840

Sperlich B, Born DP, Swarén M, Kilian Y, Geesmann B, Kohl-Bareis M, Holmberg HC (2013) Is leg compression beneficial for alpine skiers? BMC Sports Sci Med Rehabil 5(1):18

Yu G, Jang YJ, Kim J, Kim JH, Kim HY, Kim K, Panday SB (2016) Potential of IMU sensors in performance analysis of professional alpine skiers. Sensors (Basel) 16(4):463

Chapter 4
Epidemiology of Alpine Skiing Injuries

Marco Freschi

Abstract In this chapter you can find an overview of the alpine ski injuries in general population and in top athletes of different countries; differences between the two groups, identification of risk factors and mechanism of injury are analysed. We will show epidemiology in both sex, body district involved and trauma mechanisms, we highlight changes in injury numbers during last 30 years; this can be important to understand why the incidence of injuries from the 1970s to the present day significantly reduced and to learn the role that changes in safety regulations, preparation of the slopes, technical capacity of practitioners and evolution of the equipment had had in this trend. We will find that the knee is involved in more or less 50% of total alpine ski injuries. That's the reason why lower leg biomechanics is the most studied by physiologist, orthopaedics, sports physician, physiotherapist and athletic trainers that work in alpine ski in order to define injury prevention strategies.

Very few examples of articles dealing with athletes' injuries can be found in scientific literature. In 2009, the Oslo Trauma Center Research Team published a study (on behalf of the FIS, Fédération Internationale de Ski) containing the most recent and complete dataset about that topic [1]. The aim of this research was to describe the effects and the reasons of injuries of World Cup skiers during the season. In order to do so, authors employed retrospective interviews with athletes from ten different nations that had participated at least at one World Cup race during 2006/2007 and 2007/2008 seasons. In this study, researchers considered "injury" as any event that occurred during races or trainings that required the intervention of the medical staff. For every injury, the authors recorded the affected body part, the type of injury, the specific diagnosis, the place and the kind of activity that the athlete was practising (race, official trials, training on snow or preseason training). Each injury seriousness has been defined depending on the days of absence from training

M. Freschi, MD
A.C. Milan Team Doctor, Milan, Italy

National Alpine Ski Team, Italian Alpine Ski Sports Physician, Milan, Italy
e-mail: marcofreschi@yahoo.com

© Springer International Publishing AG 2018   31
H. Schoenhuber et al. (eds.), *Alpine Skiing Injuries*, Sports and Traumatology,
https://doi.org/10.1007/978-3-319-61355-0_4

sessions or competitions according to the following scheme: no rest days, very little importance (1–3 days), minor importance (4–7 days), moderate importance (8–28 days) and severe importance (beyond 28 days). Authors observed an absolute injury risk of *36.7 injuries among 100 athletes per season*. This data was obtained considering every injury occurred during the competitions season. Eighty percent among these required rest days from races and trainings, and the majority of those injuries had been considered moderate or severe. The 30% of injuries, classified as severe, required a rest period from races and training beyond 28 days. As for the difference between men and women, authors underlined how the former have more chances of injuries. However, this discrepancy loses significance when considering moderate or serious injuries. The 58% of injuries involved lower limbs, especially the knees. More than the 50% of these injuries led to a month of rest for the athlete. The legs and lumbar zone (affected in severe ways only in the 4.5% of cases) come right after that. The most common diagnosis has been anterior cruciate ligament (ACL) injuries. Authors underlined that the most frequent injury types are ligament injuries (44% of all injuries), mainly knee ligaments, followed by fractures (18%). Furthermore, in order to find a correlation between injuries and risk exposure, the authors have also calculated the relative injury risk. This rate can be found comparing the number of injuries occurred during competitions or official trainings (downhill trials) and the number of races or official trainings itself. The result has been of 9.8 injuries each 1000 runs.

A few years earlier, the French National Alpine Ski Team medical staff carried out another research [2] considering only the most frequent injury, i.e. anterior cruciate ligament injuries (as underlined by previous studies).

In 2007, in fact, Chambat published the results of an observational study conducted on the alpine skiing French national team for 25 years—from 1980 to 2005—counting 379 athletes (188 women, 191 men) that participated to a total of 1836 competitions during at least an entire season [2]. The study found 157 ACL ruptures, corresponding to an incidence of 8.5 of ACL injuries every 100 racing seasons. The incidence of the primary ACL lesion showed no significant difference in both sexes, whereas the average athletes' age at the time of the accident was significantly lower in women than men (20 ± 3.8 vs. 22 ± 3.9). Globally, more than four athletes each year have had an ACL primary lesion, and 25% of the examined athletes have suffered of at least one ACL injury throughout their career. Career length was not affected by the cruciate rupture, and no significant differences were observed in the incidence of ACL injuries in association with various disciplines of alpine skiing (slalom skiing, giant slalom, super G and downhill). Finally, the author wanted to underline that ACL injury rate within top-rank athletes (i.e. the 30 world's best skiers) is much higher than within other athletes. At least a 50% among them had suffered an ACL lesion, as well as a bilateral lesion relapse. Furthermore, the athletes in this group had longer agonistic careers compared with the others, whether they had suffered an ACL lesion or not.

From 1985 to 2014, the epidemiological archive of the Italian Winter Sports Federation (FISI) monitored more than 1000 athletes involved in competitive alpine skiing (personal data, not yet published, of Dr. M. Freschi, Dr. A. Panzeri and

Prof. Schoenhuber). The results highlighted some 900 accidents, whose 50% was localized to the knee, confirming the ACL injury as the most frequent locomotor apparatus injury, including those related to the practice of competitive alpine skiing.

According to the FISI archive data for the season 2009/2010, the incidence of ACL rupture in the 150 athletes competing in alpine ski racing season was 0.023 per 1000 h race/training athlete, considering 1500 h average time spent by the athlete every season in racing and training. Archives of football (Serie A) and rugby (national team) medical commissions have shown that in 2009/2010 season, ACL injury rate was, respectively, 0.016 and 0.049.

Technicians and medical staff following different World Cup teams observed that the most common injuries may vary depending on the competition characteristics: speed or technique [3].

In speed races, e.g. downhill and super-G, corners are wide and widely set. In this way, athletes can reach really high speed, even higher than 130 km/h. The proper race consists in a single run of about 1 min and 30 s; in downhill competitions, it is compulsory for athletes to realize at least one fast time trial before racing. In technical races, e.g. slalom and giant slalom, skiers may not reach that high speed (about 70–80 km/h), but corners are much closer, and turn radius is much tighter. Moreover, each run's length is shorter, around 50–55 s; however, the final standing is drafted considering the sum of two race times on the same slope but with different tracks [4].

Researchers observed that in speed races, due to high-speed crashes, injuries are mostly general. Fractures and head injuries are more frequent than in other disciplines [3].

Another typical injury is ACL tearing due to a wrong landing after a jump, a traditional obstacle of these speed disciplines. To perform a perfect jump, an athlete must reduce airtime for two main reasons: first of all, during airtime skis face a great deal of friction, and athletes may lose lots of speed; and then, the more the airtime, the easier it gets for the athlete to lose control of the situation, land badly and risk an injury. In order to avoid these problems during a grade change, the athlete must maintain the body's centre of mass as forward as possible, advancing the pelvis and arms. If this does not happen (usually due to fear), the jump's parabola gets higher instead of longer. Landing is another really important phase: the athlete must lean forward, absorb the impact with the snow flexing hips and knees and ensure good ground adaptation [3]. Analysing some clips taken from downhill races and computerized reconstructions, some authors have concluded that during landing athletes must deal with a 1350 N force, really close to the ligament's breaking point (between 1250 and 2500 N) [2, 5, 6]. If the athlete lands out of balance backwards, with straight knees, the tibia violently slides forward, extremely stressing the ACL (boot-top fracture or steep landing mechanism) (Fig. 4.1). Furthermore, if the jump parabola becomes too long, the athlete may land where the ground gets levelled. In this way, it is almost impossible for the athlete to absorb the impact, and he/she gets exposed to a greater risk of injury.

In technical races, however, due to lower speed and closer corners, isolated and specific lesions (e.g. sprains) are the most frequent injuries. As mentioned before,

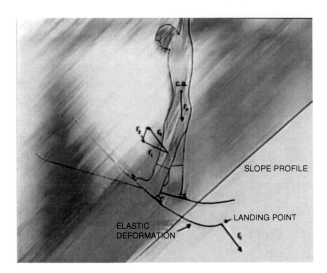

Fig. 4.1 Steep landing

knee injuries are the most common ones and usually are caused by skiers' mistakes during corners [3].

Skis used nowadays in competitions are called "carving": they have a default curve radius that depends from skis' length and carving. To steer, it is therefore enough to heel the skis on one edge or another, depending on the direction (edge inversion) [3, 7]. A valgus loading of the knee, associated with a tibial external rotation, may be caused by a mistake in the previous movement (e.g. if the athlete loads the ski on the wrong edge). Inconveniences with skis' carvings can be considered as the most common cause of knee sprains and lesions to its own ligaments [8, 9] (Fig. 4.2).

Notable efforts in the prevention of accidents related to alpine skiing have allowed a gradual decrease in accidents related to such activities over the years. The identification of safety rules that regulate skiers behaviour, a more careful preparation of the slopes and the evolution of the equipment and athletic training have resulted in a reduction of injury incidence of approximately 50% from the 1970s to today [10].

The evolution of bindings and boots turned out to be really effective in the prevention of leg fractures and ankle sprains [11, 12]. At the same time, however, the progressive increase of rigidity and height of boots alongside with the evolution of the sidecut of the ski (useful for the improvement of the performances) have determined an increase of the torsional stress to the knee which, being the first axis of free rotation above the ski, is located in a particular vulnerable biomechanical situation.

Nowadays, the knee is in fact the skeletal muscle district most frequently involved by traumas both in competitive and amateur skiers [13]. In particular, the ACL complete tear has doubled its incidence since the 1970s, and it represents 10% of all

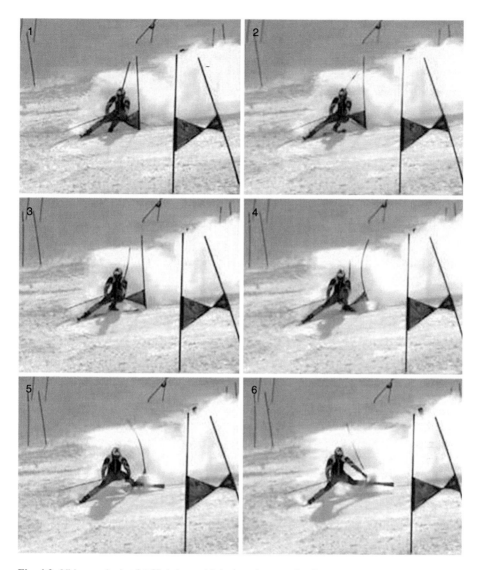

Fig. 4.2 Video analysis of ACL injury with knee valgus mechanism

injuries related to alpine skiing, resulting to be the injury most commonly associated with the practice of these sports [14, 15].

Researchers recognized that traumatic mechanisms are sometimes "boot induced", i.e. associated with the characteristics of boots. In some phases of the athletic gesture, when the athlete's centre of gravity gets backwards, the boot determines a front sliding of the tibia that may cause an ACL traumatic injury through a forced anterior drawer mechanism. This may happen, for example, when the skier tries to recover from a backwards-unbalanced position in order to prevent a fall.

With his/her hips below the level of the knees, and the ankles blocked by boots' rigidity, the only way to recover a balanced position is through a concentric quadriceps contraction. The combination of these two elements results in a forced drawer mechanism of the knee that can break the ACL, and it is known as *falling back recovery injury* [8, 9] (Fig. 4.3).

In recent years, some authors have identified another ACL lesion mechanism, called "slip-catch mechanism" [16, 17], characterized by a valgus stress/internal rotation of the knee.

The most delicate moment in a direction shift is between halfway and three-quarters of the corner, after passing the maximum descent grade [3, 7]. Indeed, in this moment, the athlete has to oppose great forces, i.e. his own acceleration and the gravity acceleration (dragging the athlete towards the end of the slope along the line of maximum grade), the centrifugal force (that pushes him/her away from the axis of rotation) and the skis' friction on the snow. In order to do so, it requires an incredibly strong quadriceps contraction, first eccentric and then isometric, even stronger on the external ski during a direction shift. If this does not happen, and the core and thigh muscles cannot bear all that effort, the athlete's centre of mass gets lower and further back, moving the load away from the ski front. The athlete may seem to be gaining a lot of speed, but that is just an illusion caused by the skis vibrating and losing grip with the snow. In this situation, slowing down may be really hard, while, at the same time, it may get really easy to lose control of the skis, rising the chances of an injury through the so-called *phantom foot* [8, 9, 18, 19] mechanism.

Furthermore, the carving ski structure does not allow the athlete to regain the correct position after a cornering mistake. The elastic distortion of the ski during cornering is consequential to skier acceleration, the gravity acceleration, the centrifugal force and the skis' friction on the snow. When these forces fail after a cornering mistake, the ski suddenly gets back to its default position, and the athlete gets thrown to the ground with the so-called spring effect [3], typical of these disciplines.

Understanding the traumatic mechanism behind an ACL tearing is a key factor to prevent these injuries. A detailed analysis of the accident is nowadays possible: thanks to the images recorded during an athlete's performance, each instant of the injury can be easily reconstructed and investigated [16, 20]. Given the great epidemiological impact of ACL injury in association with alpine skiing, the prevention of such injury remains an objective of primary importance.

Epidemiological studies, together with the analysis of the traumatic mechanisms, have been used by many national federations in coordination with the International Ski Federation (FIS) to identify specific risk factors for ACL injuries and to plan adequate prevention strategies. Knee joint kinematics studies play a particularly important role as a preventive measure to identify risk factors associated with the continuous evolution of alpine skiing equipment [21]. Thanks to these studies, the FIS has been able to provide specific directions (e.g. about the distance of the boot from the snow, the curvature radius and length of skis) that allowed a progressive decrease of ACL injuries after a period, from 1997 to 1999 in which, due to the introduction of carving skis, the ACL injury rate had been increasing terribly.

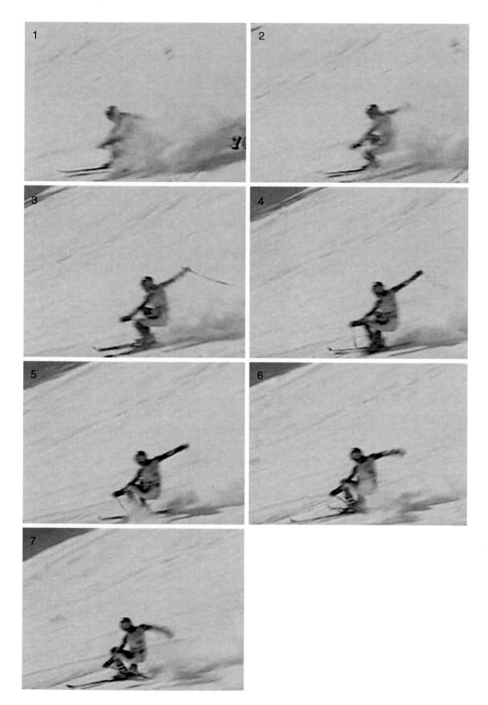

Fig. 4.3 Falling back recovery

Considering upper limb injuries, one of the most common is shoulder dislocation. As a matter of fact, to maintain a trajectory as close as possible to the gate, the athlete must knock it down with the arm opposite to cornering direction. During this movement, the inner arm may pass through the gate, stressing the glenohumeral joint with abduction and external rotation. This circumstance may occur even when placing badly the arm during falls [3].

Finally, lesions to the ulnar collateral ligament of the thumb should be included among isolated and specific lesions in skiing. This ligament is involved if the hand holding the stick hits the ground when falling [3].

For some years, alpine skiing trainers and medical staff of various national teams have been noticing an increasing number of problems and injuries which may be qualified as "wear and tear". These problems, often chronic, may heavily affect trainings and race results; on the other hand, they rarely force the athletes to stop their activity [3].

Low back pain is definitely the most common injury in this category. It may vary in traits and intensity, from a simple annoyance to an almost disabling pain that may stop the athlete and that requires specific treatments [3]. Many authors suggest that spine anomalies and lesions are caused by very common circumstances in alpine skiing, i.e. thoracolumbar spine traumas and excessive loads on this anatomical region, especially in flexed positions [22, 23]. However, international scientific literature contains very few articles dealing with the low back pain problem between skiers. Only two articles about that issue have been written, but they only analyse the problem between youngsters [24, 25].

In the more interesting one, authors compared the lumbar spine x-rays of kids, aged 11–17, who practised winter sports (alpine skiing, cross-country skiing and ski-jumping) with those of youngsters of the same age who did not practise any sport at élite levels [24]. Researchers found out that 56 kids of 120 of the "skier group" showed spine anomalies: lesions to the vertebral end plate (mainly its anterior section), degenerative disc diseases, protrusions and hernias. In the control group, individuals with anomalies were only 7 of 39. Looking at the alpine skiing young athletes specifically (77), an impressive 37 kids (almost one in two children) show anomalies to the thoracolumbar spine, especially lesions to the vertebral anterior end plate. Even the number of anomalies within the same subject is really different between the two groups: in winter-sport-practising kids, it varies from 1 to 8 within the same subject, with an average of 4, and in the remaining group, each subject may show 1 or 2 lesions.

Another article, published by Scandinavian authors, analysed overuse injuries and lumbar pain problems in a group of teenagers attending a specific ski high school. Authors highlighted that the knees and the spine are the most commonly affected parts, above all, in kids engaged in sports [25]. As a matter of fact, FIS itself published a brief pamphlet, drafted by a Canadian team member, in which readers can find the five most important ways to prevent back pain in athletes [4]. These are, however, general behavioural rules that showed how to prevent back pain within the population. They cannot be considered specific rules for alpine skiing.

References

1. Florenes TW, Bere T, Nordsletten L, Heir S, Bahr R (2009) Injuries among male and female World Cup alpine skiers. Br J Sports Med 43:973–978
2. Pujol N, Rousseaux Blanchi MP, Chambat P (2007) The incidence of anterior cruciate ligament injuries among competitive alpine skiers: a 25-year investigation. Am J Sports Med 35:1070–1074
3. Italian Alpine Ski Team technicians and trainers personal communications
4. www.fis-ski.com
5. Fischer JF, Leyvraz PF, Bally A (1994) A dynamic analysis of the knee ligament injuries in alpine skiing. Acta Orthop Belg 60:194–203
6. Genitsen KG, Nachbauer W, Van Den Bogert A (1996) Computer simulation of landing movement in downhill skiing: anterior cruciate ligament injuries. J Biomech 29:845–854
7. Cotelli C, Canclini A, Lupotto P (20–21 ottobre 2000) Analisi biomeccanica della forza espressa in curva. Atti del Secondo Congresso "La medicina dello sport e gli sport invernali": "Lo sci alpino: valutazione funzionale, tecniche di preparazione, aspetti fisiopatologici". Cuneo
8. Hunter RE (1999) Skiing injuries. Am J Sports Med 27(3):381–389
9. Koele MS, Lloyd-Smith R, Taunton JE (2002) Alpine ski injuries and their prevention. Sports Med 32(12):785–793
10. Duncan JB, Hunter R, Purnell M, Freeman J (1995) Meniscal injuries associated with anterior cruciate ligament tears in alpine skiers. Am J Sports Med 23:170–172
11. Elmqvist LG, Johnson RJ (1994) The crucial ligaments: diagnosis and treatment of ligamentous injuries about the knee. Churchill Livingstone, New York, NY, pp 495–505
12. Natri A, Beynnon BD, Ettlinger CF, Johnson RJ, Shealy JE (1999) Alpine ski bindings and injuries. Sports Med 28:35–48
13. Fu FH (2001) Sports injuries. Cap 32. Lippincott Williams & Wilkins, Baltimore
14. PL M, McQudlen EN, Eaton LA et al (1998) Downhill Ski fatalities: the Vermont experience. J Trauma 28:95
15. Marshall JL, Warren RF, Wickiewicz TL (1982) Primary surgical treatment of anterior cruciate ligament lesions. Am J Sports Med 10:103–107
16. Reid RC, Senner V, Bahr R et al (2011) Mechanisms of anterior cruciate ligament injury in world cup alpine skiing: a systematic video analysis of 20 cases. Am J Sports Med 39:1421–1429
17. Bere T, Førenes T, Krosshaug T et al (2011) Events leading to anterior cruciate ligament injury in World Cup Alpine Skiing: a systematic video analysis of 20 cases. Br J Sports Med 45:1294–1302
18. Deibert MC, Aronsson DD, Johnson RJ, Ettlinger CF (1998) Skiing injuries in children, adolescent and adults. J Bone Joint Surg 80(1):25–32
19. Ettlinger CF, Johnson RJ, Sheavy JE (1995) A method to help reduce the risk of serious knee sprains incurred in alpine skiing. Am J Sports Med 23(5):531–537
20. Bere T, Førenes T, Krosshaug T (2014) A systematic video analysis of 69 injury cases in World Cup alpine skiing. Scand J Med Sci Sports 24:667–677
21. Zorko M, Nemec B, Babic J et al (2015) The waist width of skis influences the kinematics of the knee joint in alpine skiing. J Sports Sci Med 14:606–619
22. Commandre FA, Gagnerie G, Zakarian M (1988) The child, the spine and sport. J Sports Med Phys Fitness 28:11–19
23. Sward L, Eriksson B, Peterson L (1990) Anthropometric characteristics, passive hip flexion, and spinal mobility in relation to back pain in athletes. Spine 15:376–382
24. Rachbauer F, Sterzinger W, Eibl G (2001) Radiographic abnormalities in the toracolumbar spine of young elite skiers. Am J Sports Med 29(4):446–449
25. Bergstrom KA, Brandseth K, Fretheim S, Tvilde K, Ekeland A (2004) Back injuries and pain in adolescents attending a ski high school. Knee Surg Sports Traumatol Arthrosc 12:80–85

Chapter 5
Concussion in Alpine Ski

Zefferino Rossini, Francesco Costa, Alessandro Ortolina, Massimo Tomei, Maurizio Fornari, and Valentina Re

Abstract Head injuries are a serious problem in every sports. Despite the injury prevention efforts, concussion does not decrease in frequency and they can have serious consequences. This is why it is very important to know them, recognize them, and be able to manage them.

5.1 Introduction

The number of sports-related concussions has been increasing in the last decade, likely due to a rising awareness and, thus, recognition of this pathology but also because of a higher power and strength of our athletes. In 2007, Hootman and colleagues analyzed data of the National Collegiate Athletic Association (NCAA) from 1988 to 2004 regarding all injuries, including concussion. There was no significant change in overall rate of injury; however, concussions increased significantly over this interval. In ski-related sports, head injury results the main cause for patient referral to trauma centers, and it is the major cause of morbidity and death in traumatic skiing accidents. Although the improvement in skiing equipment has led to a drop in the number of injuries in the last three decades, head injuries were an exception, since they increased during this period [1].

The role of helmets in preventing traumatic brain injury (TBI) is widely accepted. Some authors clearly indicate that helmet can be useful mainly in preventing concussion. On the other side, the efficacy of helmets in preventing moderate to severe brain injury is still debated [2–4].

Z. Rossini • F. Costa • A. Ortolina • M. Tomei • M. Fornari
Division of Neurosurgery, Humanitas Clinical and Research Center, Via Alessandro Manzoni, 56, Rozzano, MI, Italy
e-mail: fornari.maurizio@yahoo.it; maurizio.fornari@yahoo.it

V. Re (✉)
Division of Orthopaedic Rehabilitation, Galeazzi Research Hospital, Via Riccardo Galeazzi, 4, Milan, MI, Italy
e-mail: valentinare.doc@gmail.com

© Springer International Publishing AG 2018   41
H. Schoenhuber et al. (eds.), *Alpine Skiing Injuries*, Sports and Traumatology,
https://doi.org/10.1007/978-3-319-61355-0_5

The critical issues in the concussion management among skiers and snowboarders include making the diagnosis, differentiating concussion/mild traumatic brain injury (TBI) from moderate to severe TBI, recognizing any factors which may conduct to complications or may have an influence on recovery, setting a good rehabilitation protocol, and therefore determining when the patient can safely return to competition.

5.2   Epidemiology of Concussion in Skiers and Snowboarders

Unfortunately no source is available on ski-related concussion rate, and no differentiation is made between concussion/mild TBI and moderate/severe TBI, in terms of incidence.

Literature finds out that TBI is the leading cause of death in skiers and snowboarders.

Depending on the sources, the incidence of TBI ranges from 3% in France to 11% in Switzerland and 15% in the United States. In Northern America in the past decade, approximately 40 people have died per year on average during skiing and snowboarding. According to the National Sporting Goods Association, the per-participant skier/snowboarder fatality rate was 3.9 per one million on-slope participants in 2008. Despite the overall rate of reported alpine ski injuries declined slightly from 2.66 injuries per 1000 skiers in 1990 to 2.63 injuries per 1000 skiers in 2001, in snowboarding, the rate of injuries doubled from 3.37 injuries per 1000 in 1990 to 6.97 per 1000 snowboarders in 2001.

Incidence could vary for discipline and gender, but there is no consensus in literature, regarding gender prevalence in winter sport-related concussion. Epidemiologic studies taken from other sports, as in soccer, for example, revealed a higher risk for concussion in girls than in boys. It can be explained looking at the differences in biomechanics and in playing style between genders. Steenstrup et al. compared freestyle skiers and snowboarders participating to the World Cup, in a 7-year study, and he found that freestyle skiers had the highest overall head injury incidence and, across all disciplines, the injury incidence was higher in women than in men [5]. Another prospective study of head injuries in skiers and snowboarders in Japan, between 1994 and 1999, reported that snowboard-related head injuries occurred at a rate of 6.33 per 100,000 snowboarders, compared with a rate of 1.03 in skiers. The injuries were also more prevalent in males (63% of all injuries) than in women (51%) in the snowboarder group [6]. In 2015, Haaland et al. reported that among elite alpine, freestyle skiers, and snowboarders, injury incidence seems to be higher in women than in men [7], in contrast with the Japan study mentioned before.

Finally children may be more prone to head trauma than adults. Among them, a higher rate of scalp calvarial fracture has been reported.

The updated epidemiological data for elite skiers and snowboarders come from FIS (International Ski Federation) Injury Surveillance System 2006–2016 [8]. According to this report, the majority of injuries occurs during training sessions (51.9%) and not during the game, independently from the type of injury.

Among injuries, concussion accounts from 7.2% in Alpine Skiing World Cup to 12.6% in alpine skiing [8]. In 32% of cases, player returned to play after more than 28 days. However, data correlating the severity of head trauma to the absence from playing are missing.

5.3 What Is a Concussion?

Glasgow Coma Scale (GCS) score is the most widely employed classification of head trauma. It divides head trauma into *mild* (GCS 14–15), *moderate* (GCS 9–13), and *severe* (≤ 8).

Concussion is a mild head trauma; it is defined as a clinical syndrome in which a biomechanical force from a non-penetrating head injury, via acceleration-deceleration or rotational forces, transiently disrupts normal brain function, causing an alteration of consciousness without structural damage. Alteration of consciousness is not necessarily loss of consciousness (LOC), but may include only confusion and/or amnesia and/or emotional changes. Common early signs and symptoms of concussion are listed in Table 5.1.

Usually, consciousness alterations are brief, but no consensus is present in literature about the length and the duration of this event. Recovery from concussion means improvement in symptoms and in damaged skills.

The clinical findings can be explained as a transient disturbance in neuronal function which can persist up to 7–10 days after the injury, due to a hyperglycolytic and hypermetabolic state related to increased levels of intracellular glutamate, altered blood flow, and mitochondrial dysfunction [9]. During this period, the brain is more susceptible to second impacts (see below "second impact syndrome"). With the current technology, no microscopic or gross parenchymal changes can be found, and standard neuroimaging is typically normal [10, 11]. Despite that in clinical

Table 5.1 Sign and symptoms of concussion

Symptoms	Headache, dizziness, "feeling in a fog"
Physical signs	Loss of consciousness, vacant expression, vomiting, inappropriate playing behaviour, unsteady on legs, slowed reactions
Behavioural changes	Inappropriate emotions, irritability, feeling nervous or anxious
Cognitive impairment	Slowed reaction times, confusion/disorientation, poor attention and concentration, loss of memory for events up to and/or after the concussion
Sleep disturbance	Drowsiness

Table 5.2 Modifying factors that can influence concussion management

Symptoms	Severity: duration >10 days
Signs	Loss of consciousness >1 min and/or amnesia >1 min
Sequelae	Concussive convulsions
Temporal	Repeated concussions over time New injuries during time Recovery time Recent concussion or traumatic brain injury
Threshold	Concussions occurring with progressively lower impact force Slower recovery time after each concussion
Age	Child (<10 years) and adolescent (10–18 years)
Co- and pre-morbidities	Migraine, depression or other mental health disorders, attention deficit hyperactivity disorder (ADHD), learning disabilities, sleep disorders
Medication	Psychoactive drugs, anticoagulants
Behaviour	Dangerous style of play
Sport	High risk activity, contact and collision sport, high sport level

practice, it is common to perform a brain CT scan in a patient that sustained a head trauma, early imaging is not recommended if symptoms are suggestive of a concussion or a mild TBI and the patient recovers rapidly. However, if symptoms or alteration of consciousness persist, a brain CT scan is strongly suggested to exclude moderate or severe head injuries.

5.3.1   Modifying Factors that Can Influence Concussion Management

Modifying factors (listed in Table 5.2) may influence the diagnosis and the management of concussion, including intensity of symptoms, recovery time, and when return to play. In some cases they may predict if the patient will experience worse symptoms or prolonged recover.

For example, motion sickness has been recognized to be a risk factor for suffering worse balance problem and dizziness, and history of migraine will lead to worse headache [12, 13].

5.3.2   Concussion Grading

Some authors create a concussion grading system, the most famous are the one of Cantu [14] and of the American Academy of Neurology (AAN) [15] (Table 5.3). They define a "mild concussion," and the definition is similar in both scales, a "moderate and severe concussion," but their interpretation is

Table 5.3 Concussion grading

Grade	Cantu system	AAN system
1 (mild)	1. PTA <30 min 2. No LOC	1. Transient confusion 2. No LOC 3. Symptoms resolve in <15 min
2 (moderate)	1. LOC <5 min, or 2. PTA >30 min	As above, but symptoms last >15 min
3 (severe)	1. LOC ≥5 min or 2. PTA ≥24 h	Any LOC

LOC loss of consciousness, *PTA* posttraumatic amnesia

different. However, there is not enough evidence to prefer AAN scale or Cantu scale.

5.3.3 Second Impact Syndrome (SIS)

Following a concussive brain injury, there is a window of metabolic vulnerability, whose duration seems to last 7–10 days or more after the first impact. Second impact syndrome (SIS) was first reported in 1973 by Shneider and later in 1984 by Saunders and Harbaugh, who described massive cerebral edema after a second head injury before recovery from a first head impact. In this case report, a young football player, who suffered from a concussion during the game, returned to play 4 days later and suffered an additional head trauma. This second concussion resulted in massive cerebral edema, leading to coma and to his death [16].

Nowadays SIS is well recognized and is explained as neuron death during a brain trauma that happened in a condition of metabolic vulnerability and inadequate blood flow.

Similar metabolic dysfunction findings were reported by Vagnozzi et al. among concussed athletes. Altered cerebral metabolism was documented using magnetic resonance spectroscopy imaging in concussed athletes and in those sustaining a second injury prior to resolution of the first [17, 18].

5.3.4 Post-concussion Syndrome

It refers to a collection of symptoms that last more than 3–6 months. Controversies exist about the contribution of organic dysfunction versus psychological factors. Symptoms frequently observed in this syndrome are somatic, cognitive, and psychological. Many patients complain of headache, described as mild to moderate, which could be tension type and refractory to pharmacologic treatment. Dizziness and memory difficulties are the most common symptoms. Expert management is warranted for post-concussion syndrome.

5.4   Mechanism of Head Injury and Risk Factors Among Snowboarders and Skiers

Until now, no worldwide study about the mechanism of concussion and risk factors associated with winter sports has been conducted. The majority of informations come from single or multicenter studies or national archives focused on the TBI mechanism in winter sports. From the available data, some considerations can be listed:

- Differences in mechanism of head injury between skiers and snowboarders are weak.
- Environmental factors play a pivotal role in traumatic skiing and snowboarding injuries.
- There is lack of homogeneity in data collection (medical service, retrospective telephone survey, ski patrol).
- Injury assessment and patient management can differ from organization between elite skiers and recreational skiers.

Despite that speed, slope types, skiers' experience, and slope crowding can reasonably be considered as risk factors for mild TBI, they are under-reported in literature and seem not to be crucial in influencing the rate and type of head injury. Collecting this kind of information in an emergency department is really difficult, and it is likely to be the explanation to the lack of data.

Advances in skiing/snowboarding techniques and equipment have unavoidably produced increased velocities and jumping heights. Collisions can occur with other participants or with objects. The best way to promote a prevention program is, first of all, to emphasize to follow a responsible behavior.

In a paper of January 2017, Bailly et al. investigated the mechanisms leading to head trauma in a cohort of 295 skiers and 71 snowboarders; they found that falls account for the majority of head trauma mechanisms (54%), collision with an obstacle caused the more serious TBI, and falling on the head is a frequent type of fall. The latter statement can be, respectively, explained for snowboarders with the "opposite edge phenomenon" (described as the edge of the snowboard catching in the snow in a direction opposite to the direction of the turn, causing a sudden stop and the projection of the upper body against the slope) and for skiers with crossing skis. According to their findings, the most frequent pattern of injury leading to mild TBI or concussion is falling. Finally, they divided three categories of patients in relation to head trauma causes: men aged 16–26 years are more prone to be involved in crash at high speed or in connection with jumps; beginners, women, and children aged <16 years frequently experience collisions between users; skiers older than 50 years usually are non-helmeted and are frequently involved in falls [19].

Different findings were reported by Levy et al. Among skiers and snowboarders of all ages admitted to an emergency department for head injury, they noticed that skier-tree collision was the most common mechanism of head trauma [20].

In addition, a risk factor referred by Baschera is skiing off-piste: it seems that it is linked to a seven- to eightfold higher risk for sustaining moderate and severe TBI in recreational skiers [21].

5.5   The Role of Helmet in Preventing Concussion

A separate discussion is needed for winter sport helmets. As introduced above, the helmet use in skiing and snowboarding is commonly considered a protective factor against TBI, mainly mTBI. Helmets can act through three mechanisms:

1. Minimize the acceleration-deceleration injury.
2. Spread the impact over a larger surface area.
3. Protect the head and skull from direct impact.

While the efficacy of helmets in preventing head injury has been clearly proved for motorcyclists and cyclists, results are not so clear for skiers and snowboarders [22–25].

Hagel and Sulheim have independently described in case control studies, respectively, conducted in Canada and Norway, an incidence reduction of TBI in subjects wearing helmets [3, 4]. Mueller confirmed their observation, finding a major benefit in younger subjects [26]. In a systematic review, Cusimano reported a reduction in the risk of head injury with helmet use ranging from 15% to 60% [27].

Conversely, Baschera et al. conducted a cohort study investigating the association between head injury and helmet use in alpine skiers in a tertiary trauma center from 2000–2001 to 2010–2011. The results of the authors showed an increased helmet use during this decade (from 0% to 71%), but no decrease in the incidence of both mild TBI and moderate to severe TBI [21]. Recently, Bergmann et al. conducted a retrospective analysis evaluating if the helmet use could influence the rate of concussion among young skiers and snowboarders: the results were similar to those reported by Baschera et al., i.e., the rate of mild TBI was similar in helmet users compared to non-helmet users [28].

In order to clarify the role of helmets in head injury prevention and to suggest valid recommendation about the helmet use in recreational skiers and snowboarders, an evidence-based review by Haider et al. established that *all recreational skiers and snowboarders should wear safety helmets to reduce the incidence and severity of head injury during these sports* (level I recommendation). Helmet use does not seem to increase the risk compensation behavior and the risk of cervical spine injuries. According to this, the policies and intervention directed toward promoting helmet use should be supported to reduce mortality and morbidity [29].

However, the role of confounding factors like skiing experience, elite versus recreational skiers, and speed or quality of the equipment is neither always taken into account nor easy to investigate. Without adjustment of data referred to helmet use with these confounding factors, despite the evidences reported in literature, it is difficult to establish the real power of helmet use in TBI prevention.

Table 5.4 Helmet safety standards

	CEN 1077	ASTM F2040
Single drop height	1.5 m	2.0 m, with a peak velocity of 6.2 m/s
Peak acceleration on headform	Must not exceed 250 Gs upon impact	Must not exceed 300 Gs upon impact
Impact energy called for	69 J	98 J
Testing temperature range specified for ski helmets	None	Low: −22 to −28 °C, high: 32 to 38°C Tests carried out in cold, hot and wet conditions
Penetration test	"Drop-hammer" test	None
Retention system (chin strap) test	Included	Dynamic strength retention test

While adult recreational skiers are not obliged by specific law to wear a helmet during skiing or snowboarding, different rules have to be followed by elite professionals.

The crash helmets recommended by FIS for alpine ski events are compulsory at all FIS alpine ski events and should satisfy the following safety standards [30]:

– For *giant slalom, super-G,* and *downhill,* the helmet model has to fulfill and to be certified under both ASTM 2040 and EN 1077 (class A). In addition helmet model has to pass an additional specific test under EN 1077 test procedure but at higher test speed of 6.8 m/s.
– For *slalom,* helmet model has to be certified under EN 1077 (class B) or ASTM 2040 as minimum standards. Crash helmets fulfilling higher safety standards can be used a fortiori in slalom. This includes EN 1077 (class A), SNELL 98, and all helmets fulfilling the giant slalom-, super-G-, and downhill-specific standard described above. Before being on sale, each helmet needs to be tested according to American Society for Testing and Materials and CSN EN Standard [2, 31]. The main parameters used for testing protocols for EN 1077 and ASTM 2040 are reported in the Table 5.4.

Why the use of helmets had no significant protection for moderate to severe TBI is explained below.

The modern winter sport helmets protect people from an impact speed between 18 and 23 km/h or falls from up to 2.4 m. Ruedl et al. recorded that the average skiing speeds are about 40–48 km/h [32]. This means that also the best available helmets do not provide sufficient protection at such speed.

5.6   What Happens if a Skier Has Sustained a Concussion?

FIS Medical Guide follows the rules derived from the *consensus statement on concussion in sport held in Berlin in November 2016* [33]. The recommendation taken from the FIS has been weighted on elite professionals [34]. However, in our opinion they can be applied also in recreational skiers. Unfortunately, the organization of emergency services on slopes attended by recreational skiers cannot be as effective as for elite skiers.

The first step in case of suspected concussion is the sudden removal of the athlete from the field for a medical evaluation. The rhyme to follow in this situation is "When in doubt, sit them out." Athlete must not resume participation once removed from the slope for suspected concussion. A fast clinical examination of the athletes can be performed using the SCAT5, an easy and complete scale that has been proposed to diagnose a concussion. SCAT5 should be used by medical staff, and it includes symptoms, balance testing, memory testing, GCS score, Maddock score, cognitive state, and neck injury and delayed recall.

It takes about 10 min to be done. There is also the Child-SCAT5, which can be used for children, and the concussion recognition tool 5 (Fig. 5.1), which can be used by nonmedical staff (as coaches, race officials, fellow athletes, or physiotherapist).

If a skier fails to answer any of the memory questions correctly, or shows a lack of balance, or any of the red flag symptoms listed, or there are any concerns that the athlete is suspected of having concussion, then he/she should be definitively removed from play to avoid a second impact syndrome and referred to a medical practitioner or emergency department. Usually a CT scan is performed, and major traumatic brain injuries excluded. The athlete is then sent back to the medical team doctor.

Recovery is usually spontaneous with rapid resolution of symptoms. This could encourage the athlete to ignore concussion symptoms, exposing them to the second impact syndrome, or delay their return to play. It is not clear which number of traumatic events are needed, but we know that repeated concussions could shorten an athlete's career and may lead to permanent neurological impairment.

5.7 Rehabilitation and Return to Play

Rehabilitation is the key to a safe return to play.

It is important to collect all sign and symptoms presented the day of the injury until 1 week later. This will help clinicians to identify which functional area is involved, its gravity, and presence of personal risk factors.

With the informations collected, doctors are sometimes able to "predict recovery time." For example, R.J Elbin et al. found that a prompt removal from play is linked to a faster recovery time [35]. Kontos et al. say that personal background story of previous concussions, migraine, motion sickness, sleep problem, learning disabilities, or psychiatric disorders could determine a higher gravity of symptoms and a longer recovery time [12, 13]. Objective examination is also fundamental for recovery time: A.M. Sufrinko et al. found that post-traumatic migraine, fatigue, and eye motor speed are connected with prolonged recovery time [36, 37].

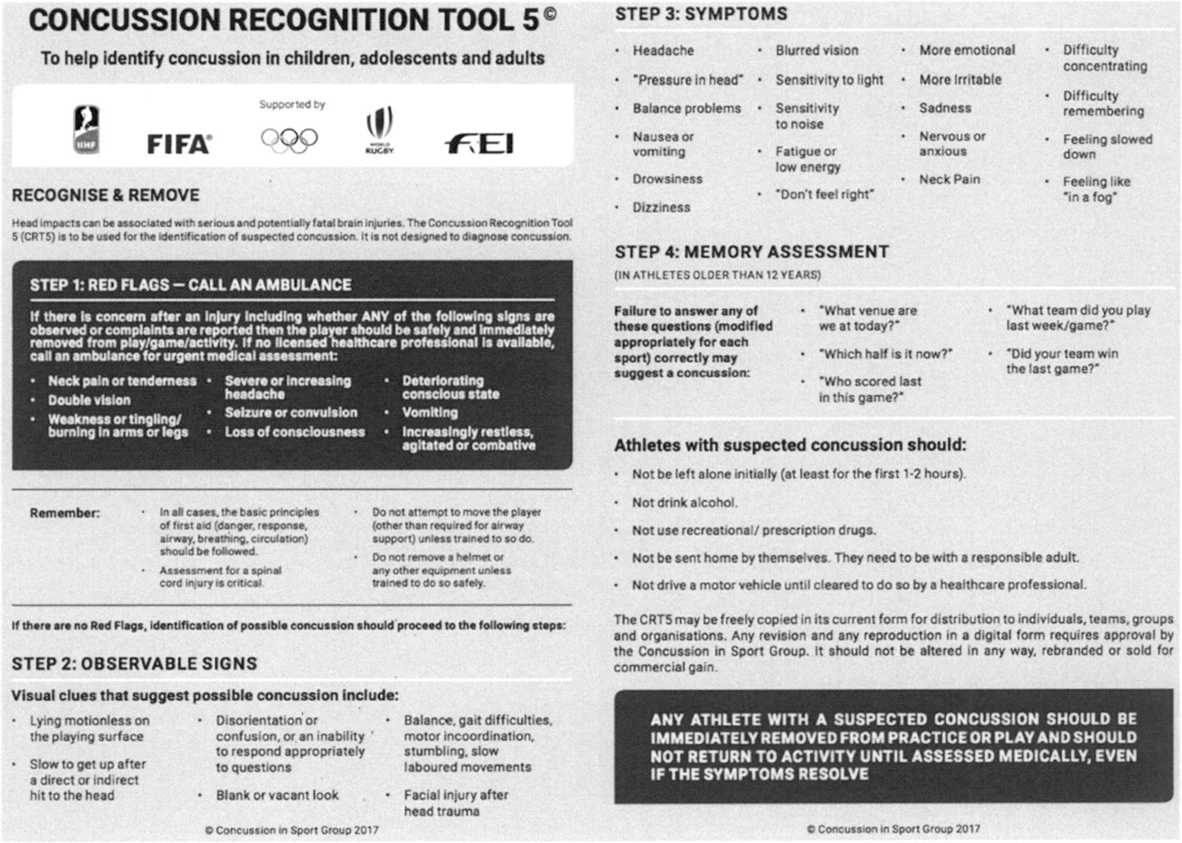

CONCUSSION RECOGNITION TOOL 5©

To help identify concussion in children, adolescents and adults

Supported by

RECOGNISE & REMOVE

Head impacts can be associated with serious and potentially fatal brain injuries. The Concussion Recognition Tool 5 (CRT5) is to be used for the identification of suspected concussion. It is not designed to diagnose concussion.

STEP 1: RED FLAGS — CALL AN AMBULANCE

If there is concern after an injury including whether ANY of the following signs are observed or complaints are reported then the player should be safely and immediately removed from play/game/activity. If no licensed healthcare professional is available, call an ambulance for urgent medical assessment:

- **Neck pain or tenderness**
- **Double vision**
- **Weakness or tingling/burning in arms or legs**
- **Severe or increasing headache**
- **Seizure or convulsion**
- **Loss of consciousness**
- **Deteriorating conscious state**
- **Vomiting**
- **Increasingly restless, agitated or combative**

Remember:

- In all cases, the basic principles of first aid (danger, response, airway, breathing, circulation) should be followed.
- Assessment for a spinal cord injury is critical.
- Do not attempt to move the player (other than required for airway support) unless trained to so do.
- Do not remove a helmet or any other equipment unless trained to do so safely.

If there are no Red Flags, identification of possible concussion should proceed to the following steps:

STEP 2: OBSERVABLE SIGNS

Visual clues that suggest possible concussion include:

- Lying motionless on the playing surface
- Slow to get up after a direct or indirect hit to the head
- Disorientation or confusion, or an inability to respond appropriately to questions
- Blank or vacant look
- Balance, gait difficulties, motor incoordination, stumbling, slow laboured movements
- Facial injury after head trauma

© Concussion in Sport Group 2017

STEP 3: SYMPTOMS

- Headache
- "Pressure in head"
- Balance problems
- Nausea or vomiting
- Drowsiness
- Dizziness
- Blurred vision
- Sensitivity to light
- Sensitivity to noise
- Fatigue or low energy
- "Don't feel right"
- More emotional
- More Irritable
- Sadness
- Nervous or anxious
- Neck Pain
- Difficulty concentrating
- Difficulty remembering
- Feeling slowed down
- Feeling like "in a fog"

STEP 4: MEMORY ASSESSMENT

(IN ATHLETES OLDER THAN 12 YEARS)

Failure to answer any of these questions (modified appropriately for each sport) correctly may suggest a concussion:

- "What venue are we at today?"
- "Which half is it now?"
- "Who scored last in this game?"
- "What team did you play last week/game?"
- "Did your team win the last game?"

Athletes with suspected concussion should:

- Not be left alone initially (at least for the first 1-2 hours).
- Not drink alcohol.
- Not use recreational/ prescription drugs.
- Not be sent home by themselves. They need to be with a responsible adult.
- Not drive a motor vehicle until cleared to do so by a healthcare professional.

The CRT5 may be freely copied in its current form for distribution to individuals, teams, groups and organisations. Any revision and any reproduction in a digital form requires approval by the Concussion in Sport Group. It should not be altered in any way, rebranded or sold for commercial gain.

ANY ATHLETE WITH A SUSPECTED CONCUSSION SHOULD BE IMMEDIATELY REMOVED FROM PRACTICE OR PLAY AND SHOULD NOT RETURN TO ACTIVITY UNTIL ASSESSED MEDICALLY, EVEN IF THE SYMPTOMS RESOLVE

© Concussion in Sport Group 2017

Fig. 5.1 Concussion recognition tool 5 (CRT5)

Based on the fifth international consensus statement on concussion in sport held in Berlin in 2016, the first intervention is "physical and cognitive rest" until the acute symptoms resolved, they should avoid non-prescribed medications (Fig. 5.2). The patient should be free of symptoms at least for 24–48 h to start any rehabilitation [38]. The rehabilitation program adopted by FIS is called "graduated return to play protocol." It consists in six different stages based on aerobic training with incremental loading exercises:

- Light aerobic exercise (70% heart rate, no resistance training)
- Sport-specific exercise (no head impact activity)
- Resistance training, coordination, cognitive load (noncontact)
- Full-contact practice (normal team training)
- Return to normal game play

It is possible to pass to the next step if no symptoms are produced at least during 24 h; otherwise the patients should stay at the same activity level [33]. Return to alpine skiing is possible if normal training and play remains symptoms free. Usually a neurological assessment is performed before returning to play. If there is no medical support during the graduated return to play protocol, a 21-day off the slope should be respected.

Usually recovery is achieved in 15–30 days in most cases, but in an average of 10% it is not [38] and will follow a longer recovery time. Vagnozzi et al. documented that an altered mitochondrial metabolism is seen during recovery time and that it could last longer than symptom resolution; therefore doctors should be careful in sending back to play a patient with altered magnetic resonance spectroscopy imaging [17, 18].

Rehabilitation stage	Functional exercise at each stage of rehabilitation	Objective of each stage
No activity	Physical and cognitive rest	Recovery
Light aerobic exercise	Walking, swimming or stationary cycling keeping intensity, 70% maximum predicted heart rate. No resistance training	Increase heart rate
Sport-specific exercise	Skating drills in ice hockey, running drills in soccer. No head impact activities	Add movement
Non-contact training drills	Progression to more complex training drills, eg passing drills in football and ice hockey. May start progressive resistance training	Exercise, coordination, and cognitive load
Full contact practice	Following medical clearance participate in normal training activities	Restore confidence and assess functional skills by coaching staff
Return to play	Normal game play	

Fig. 5.2 Consensus statement on concussion in sport: the Fifth International Conference on Concussion in Sport, Berlin, November 2016

5.7.1   New Perspective

The consensus statement on concussion in sport of 2016 differs from the previous because it introduces the idea of a specialized rehabilitation. It states that "if symptoms are persistent (e.g. more than 10–14 days in adults or more than 1 month in children) the athlete should be referred to a healthcare professional who is an expert in the management of concussion" [33]. It is growing the evidence that a personalized rehabilitation is the key for functional restoration and complete recovery.

Nowadays few specialized clinics are present in Europe.

How do they manage a patient with a suspected concussion? Clinical and psychological evaluation is the key to set an individualized rehabilitation protocol. They analyze type of symptoms, their gravity, and if they are worsened by the activity of daily living.

A clinical examination is performed for neurological problems, neck pain, and vestibular and oculomotor evaluation. Collins et al. create VOMS (vestibular/ocular motor screening), an easy and rapid screening for these issues. It consists in asking the patient to do different tasks as rapid eye movement, rapid head movement, and eye convergence and then to verify a worsening in symptoms reported [39, 40].

Concussion symptoms are usually worsened by exercise; thus a complete examination requires also an exertional test which helps making the diagnosis and setting a threshold where exercise becomes symptomatic [41, 42] (Fig. 5.3). Finally a neuropsychological test is performed to understand cognitive and psychological impairments. No consensus is present in literature about which test should be done, and many protocols have been proposed [43].

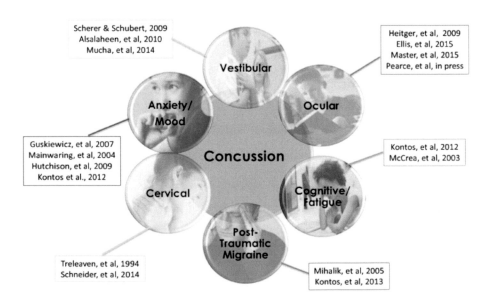

Fig. 5.3 A comprehensive, targeted approach to the clinical care of athletes following sport-related concussion. Collins MW et al. Knee Surg Sports Traumatol Arthrosc. 2014 Feb

Based on this examination, experts can differentiate six different types of concussion symptoms:

- Cognitive and fatigue
- Anxiety and mood alteration
- Migraine
- Vestibular
- Ocular
- Cervical

From this baseline, experts will set a specific treatment: for example, neck pain will be treated with passive mobilization, massage, and muscle relaxant; vestibular dysfunction should be managed by a specialized therapist with vestibular stimulation exercises; ocular motor impairment will be treated with eye movement and convergence exercises; cognitive issues are treated with cognitive therapy; and so on [44–48]. This specific approach seems to be more effective on personal symptoms and on recovery time.

If symptoms becomes chronic and are not responsive to physical therapy, a pharmacological approach could help [49]. Adaptive interventions should also be taken into account: prismatic lenses are sometimes useful for convergence correction [50].

5.8 Conclusion

Concussion in skiers and snowboarders is common at all ages. The diagnosis is only clinical and can be helped by assessment tools internationally accepted like CRT and SCAT5. Despite that the introduction of helmets has drastically reduced the incidence of mild TBI, their role in preventing moderate to severe TBI remains controversial. The first rule to respect in suspected concussion is the sudden removal of the athlete from the field. Return to play can be allowed after completing the GRTP protocol, from 6 to 30 days from the injury, depending whether the patient is free of symptoms. New perspective in rehabilitation setting is promising better results and a safer return to play. Several clinical tools are required to choose the best rehabilitation program, which has to be driven by experts' recommendations, patient's individual symptoms, and evidence-based medicine. Spreading concussion awareness and following a responsibility code is a first step for concussion prevention.

References

1. Ackery A, Hagel BE, Provvidenza C, Tator CH (2007) An international review of head and spinal cord injuries in alpine skiing and snowboarding. Inj Prev 13(6):368–375
2. (CSN) EN 1077 (2007) Helmets for alpine skiers and snowboarders: European standards. http://www.en-standard.eu/csn-en-1077-helmets-for-alpine-skiers-and-snowboarders/. Accessed 27 Jan 2014

3. Hagel BE, Pless IB, Goulet C, Platt RW, Robitaille Y (2005) Effectiveness of helmets in skiers and snowboarders: case-control and case crossover study. BMJ 330(7486):281
4. Sulheim S, Ekeland A, Holme I, Bahr R (2017) Helmet use and risk of head injuries in alpine skiers and snowboarders: changes after an interval of one decade. Br J Sports Med 51(1): 44–50
5. Steenstrup SE, Bere T, Bahr R (2014) Head injuries among FIS World Cup alpine and freestyle skiers and snowboarders: a 7-year cohort study. Br J Sports Med 48(1):41–45
6. McBeth PB, Ball CG, Mulloy RH, Kirkpatrick AW (2009) Alpine ski and snowboarding traumatic injuries: incidence, injury patterns, and risk factors for 10 years. Am J Surg 197(5):560–563
7. Haaland B, Steenstrup SE, Bere T, Bahr R, Nordsletten L (2016) Injury rate and injury patterns in FIS World Cup alpine skiing (2006–2015): have the new ski regulations made an impact? Br J Sports Med 50(1):32–36
8. Oslo Sport Trauma Research Center : FIS Injury Surveillance System 2006–2016. http://www.fisski.com/mm/Document/documentlibrary/Medical/08/57/62/FIS_ISS_report_2015-16_Neutral.pdf
9. Giza CC, Hovda DA (2014) The new neurometabolic cascade of concussion. Neurosurgery 75(Suppl 4):S24–S33
10. Kamins J, Giza CC (2016) Concussion-mild traumatic brain injury: recoverable injury with potential for serious sequelae. Neurosurg Clin N Am 27(4):441–452
11. Laker SR (2015) Sports-related concussion. Curr Pain Headache Rep 19(8):41
12. Sufrinko A, Pearce K, Elbin RJ, Covassin T, Johnson E, Collins M, Kontos AP (2015) The effect of preinjury sleep difficulties on neurocognitive impairment and symptoms after sport-related concussion. Am J Sports Med 43(4):830–838
13. Covassin T, Elbin RJ, Harris W, Parker T, Kontos A (2012) The role of age and sex in symptoms, neurocognitive performance, and postural stability in athletes after concussion. Am J Sports Med 40(6):1303–1312
14. Cantu RC (1992) Cerebral concussion in sport. Management and prevention. Sports Med 14(1):64–74
15. American Academy of Neurology (1997) Practice parameter: the management of concussion in sports (summary statement): report of the quality standards subcommittee. Neurology 48:581–585
16. Saunders R, Harbaugh R (1984) The second impact in catastrophic contact-sports head trauma. JAMA 252:538–539
17. Vagnozzi R, Signoretti S, Cristofori L, Alessandrini F, Floris R, Isgro E et al (2010) Assessment of metabolic brain damage and recovery following mild traumatic brain injury: a multicentre, proton magnetic resonance spectroscopic study in concussed patients. Brain 133(11):3232–3242
18. Vagnozzi R, Signoretti S, Tavazzi B, Floris R, Ludovici A, Marziali S et al (2008) Temporal window of metabolic brain vulnerability to concussion: a pilot H-magnetic resonance spectroscopy study in concussed athletes – Part III. Neurosurgery 62(6):1286–1295
19. Bailly N, Afquir S, Laporte JD, Melot A, Savary D, Seigneuret E, Delay JB, Donnadieu T, Masson C, Arnoux PJ (2017) Analysis of injury mechanisms in head injuries in skiers and snowboarders. Med Sci Sports Exerc 49(1):1–10
20. Levy AS, Hawkes AP, Hemminger LM, Knight S (2002) An analysis of head injuries among skiers and snowboarders. J Trauma 53(4):695–704
21. Baschera D, Hasler RM, Taugwalder D, Exadaktylos A, Raabe A (2015) Association between head injury and helmet use in alpine skiers: cohort study from a Swiss level 1 trauma center. J Neurotrauma 32(8):557–562
22. Evans L, Frick MC (1988) Helmet effectiveness in preventing motorcycle driver and passenger fatalities. Accid Anal Prev 20:447–458
23. Norvell DC, Cummings P (2002) Association of helmet use with death in motorcycle crashes: a matched-pair cohort study. Am J Epidemiol 156:483–487
24. Thompson DC, Rivara FP, Thompson RS (1996) Effectiveness of bicycle safety helmets in preventing head injuries. A case-control study. JAMA 276:1968–1973

25. Thompson RS, Rivara FP, Thompson DC (1989) A case-control study of the effectiveness of bicycle safety helmets. N Engl J Med 320:1361–1367
26. Mueller BA, Cummings P, Rivara FP, Brooks MA, Terasaki RD (2008) Injuries of the head, face, and neck in relation to ski helmet use. Epidemiology 19(2):270–276
27. Cusimano MD, Kwok J (2010) The effectiveness of helmet wear in skiers and snowboarders: a systematic review. Br J Sports Med 44(11):781–786. https://doi.org/10.1136/bjsm.2009.070573
28. Bergmann KR, Flood A, Kreykes NS, Kharbanda AB (2016) Concussion among youth skiers and snowboarders: a review of the National Trauma Data Bank from 2009 to 2010. Pediatr Emerg Care 32(1):9–13
29. Haider AH, Saleem T, Bilaniuk JW, Barraco RD, Eastern Association for the Surgery of Trauma Injury Control Violence Prevention Committee (2012) An evidence-based review: efficacy of safety helmets in the reduction of head injuries in recreational skiers and snowboarders. J Trauma Acute Care Surg 73(5):1340–1347
30. FIS (September 2014) Specifications for competition equipment and commercial markings, Edition 2014/15
31. American Society for Testing and Materials (ASTM) (2011) F2040-11; Standard specification for helmets used for recreational snow sports: ASTM. www.astm.org/Standards/F2040.htm. Accessed 27 Jan 2014
32. Ruedl G, Brunner F, Woldrich T, Faulhaber M, Kopp M, Nachbauer W, Burtscher M (2013) Factors associated with the ability to estimate actual speeds in recreational alpine skiers. Wilderness Environ Med 24(2):118–123
33. P McCrory et al (2017) Consensus statement on concussion in sport—The 5th International Conference on Concussion in Sport held in Berlin, October 2016 Br J Sports Med
34. FIS Medical Guide, Edition 2013. http://www.fis-ski.com/mm/Document/documentlibrary/Medical/03/31/99/fis-medical-guide-2013_Neutral.pdf
35. Elbin RJ, Sufrinko A, Schatz P, French J, Henry L, Burkhart S, Collins MW, Kontos AP (2016) Removal from play after concussion and recovery time. Pediatrics 138(3):e20160910
36. Sufrinko AM, Marchetti GF, Cohen PE, Elbin RJ, Re V, Kontos AP (2017) Using acute performance on a comprehensive neurocognitive, vestibular, and ocular motor assessment battery to predict recovery duration after sport-related concussions. Am J Sports Med 1:363546516685061
37. Kontos AP, Elbin RJ, Lau B, Simensky S, Freund B, French J et al (2013) Posttraumatic migraine as a predictor of recovery and cognitive impairment after sport-related concussion. Am J Sports Med 41:1497–1504
38. Iverson GL, Brooks BL, Collins MW, Lovell MR (2006) Tracking neuropsychological recovery following concussion in sport. Brain Inj 20(3):245–252
39. Mucha A, Collins MW, Elbin RJ, Furman JM, Troutman-Enseki C, DeWolf RM, Marchetti G, Kontos AP (2014) A brief vestibular/ocular motor screening (VOMS) assessment to evaluate concussions: preliminary findings. Am J Sports Med 42(10):2479–2486
40. Kontos AP, Sufrinko A, Elbin RJ, Puskar A, Collins MW (2016) Reliability and associated risk factors for performance on the vestibular/ocular motor screening (VOMS) tool in healthy collegiate athletes. Am J Sports Med 44(6):1400–1406
41. McGrath N, Dinn WM, Collins MW, Lovell MR, Elbin RJ, Kontos AP (2013) Post-exertion neurocognitive test failure among student-athletes following concussion. Brain Inj 27(1):103–113
42. Leddy J, Hinds A, Sirica D, Willer B (2016) The role of controlled exercise in concussion management. PM R 8(3 Suppl):S91–S100
43. Kontos AP, Sufrinko A, Womble M, Kegel N (2016) Neuropsychological assessment following concussion: an evidence-based review of the role of neuropsychological assessment pre- and post-concussion. Curr Pain Headache Rep 20(6):38
44. Collins MW, Kontos AP, Reynolds E, Murawski CD, Fu FH (2014) A comprehensive, targeted approach to the clinical care of athletes following sport-related concussion. Knee Surg Sports Traumatol Arthrosc 22(2):235–246
45. Broglio SP, Collins MW, Williams RM, Mucha A, Kontos AP (2015) Current and emerging rehabilitation for concussion: a review of the evidence. Clin Sports Med 34(2):213–231

46. Elbin RJ, Schatz P, Lowder HB, Kontos AP (2014) An empirical review of treatment and reha-
    bilitation approaches used in the acute, sub-acute, and chronic phases of recovery following
    sports-related concussion. Curr Treat Options Neurol 16(11):320
47. Alsalaheen BA, Mucha A, Morris LO, Whitney SL, Furman JM, Camiolo-Reddy CE, Collins
    MW, Lovell MR, Sparto PJ (2010) Vestibular rehabilitation for dizziness and balance disorders
    after concussion. J Neurol Phys Ther 34(2):87–93
48. Gallaway M, Scheiman M, Mitchell GL (2017) Vision therapy for post-concussion vision dis-
    orders. Optom Vis Sci 94(1):68–73
49. Reddy CC, Collins M, Lovell M, Kontos AP (2013) Efficacy of amantadine treatment on
    symptoms and neurocognitive performance among adolescents following sports-related con-
    cussion. J Head Trauma Rehabil 28(4):260–265
50. Rosner MS, Feinberg DL, Doble JE, Rosner AJ (2016) Treatment of vertical heterophoria
    ameliorates persistent post-concussive symptoms: a retrospective analysis utilizing a multi-
    faceted assessment battery. Brain Inj 30(3):311–317

Chapter 6
Traumatic Dislocation and Fractures

Andrea Panzeri, Paolo Capitani, Gabriele Thiébat, and Herbert Schoenhuber

Abstract Alpine Ski is an high energy sport where athletes reach high speeds. Their joints are undergone to several stresses that can lead to traumas of two types: generic and specific for joints. The first one are the injuries caused by high energy traumas and usually happen more often in Downhill (DH) and Super-Giant Slalom (SG). In Giant Slalom (GS) and Slalom (SL), the joint usually undergo a specific mechanism of injury due to an inappropriate movement.

Alpine ski is a popular sport practiced worldwide by an increasing number of people, estimated at around 200,000,000 people [1]. In the United States of America (USA), from 12 to 15 millions of people went to ski every year [2, 3]. In Austria, eight million skiers were recorded in a year [4]. Other winter sports have spread and established in the recent decades slowing the diffusion of alpine skiing, such as snowboarding, but no one has ever reached the same number of athletes [1, 5] (Fig. 6.1).

Alpine ski is a high-energy sport where athletes reach high speeds. Their joints undergo several stresses that can lead to traumas of two types: generic and specific for joints. The first one are the injuries caused by high-energy traumas and usually happen more often in downhill (DH) and super-giant slalom (SG). In giant slalom (GS) and slalom (SL), the joint usually undergoes a specific mechanism of injury due to an inappropriate movement [6]. Similar traumatic mechanisms were also found in recreational ski. We are witnessing an increasing number of injuries due also to a rising spread of this sport in the general population. In many articles, the number of injuries in recreational ski is reported with the "skier days" method which gives an idea of the size of the problem [1, 7]. Recreational skiers were reported to have 3 injuries/1000 skier-days. [1, 7–9]. There were little differences depending on the population examined. In Austria, two injuries/1000 skier-days were reported [4]. In the literature, there were few data regarding injuries that

A. Panzeri • P. Capitani (✉) • G. Thiébat • H. Schoenhuber
Sport Traumatology Centre, IRCCS Istituto Ortopedico Galeazzi,
Via Riccardo Galeazzi 4, 20161 Milano, Italy
e-mail: paolocapitani.dr@gmail.com

© Springer International Publishing AG 2018
H. Schoenhuber et al. (eds.), *Alpine Skiing Injuries*, Sports and Traumatology,
https://doi.org/10.1007/978-3-319-61355-0_6

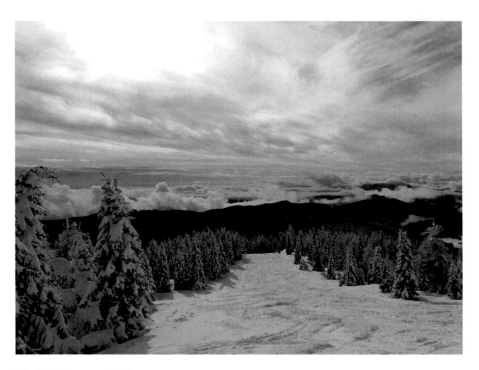

Fig. 6.1 View on a ski slope

require hospitalization and intensive care unit (ICU) admissions. Injuries with ISS > 12 are reported close to 0.06–0.07/1000 skier-days. Most of the injuries occur in the afternoon, most likely due to a worse condition of the snow and also to the onset of fatigue and reduced visibility and on slope intersections [1, 7–9]. In the ski areas, two highly risk areas of injury were slope intersections and snow parks. In slope intersections, there were a prevalence of collisions and injuries of the upper limbs mainly due to unexpected impacts. In the snow parks, there was a higher incidence of injury in younger people, but you have to take into account the prevalence of snowboarders in these areas. These two areas had injuries with different characteristics to those of injuries on the ski slopes [4]. Age, presence of soft snow, and beginner skiers are predictive factors to falls. In 10 years the incidence of falls decreased [10]. In literature, it was reported that the presence of snowboarders significantly increased the risk of injuries on the slopes compared to the same slopes only with skiers [11].

Beginners had an increased risk of injury up to seven times. Skiing instructions especially helped to prevent serious injuries [12].

In recreational skiing and in team sports, women had a greater risk of injury, but it has been shown that in professional skiing this significative difference did not occur considering knees and anterior cruciate ligament (ACL) injuries. Men had a higher risk than women of severe injuries. Therefore, men and women need an equal program of injuries prevention [13].

Tibia and fibula fractures are more frequent in children than adults and elite athletes [1, 7–9]. In the USA, around 13–27% of the recreational skiers are children, and their injury rate was reported to be 3.92–9.1/1000 skier-days [2]. Past studies report that of all injuries in four ski seasons in Norway, almost half involved children and adolescents [14].

Toward the mid-nineteenth century, skiing was exported from the Scandinavian countries to the USA. In Scandinavian countries with their history, environment, and climate, snow's sports were widespread practiced also in high school. A study analyzed the population of a Swedish ski high school and reported that the younger the athlete who suffers an injury, the easier he would have a new injury in the same, or in a new, anatomical region. About half of the students in their study period in ski high school had at least an injury. These injuries were usually classified as severe or moderate and the most part of them involved lower limbs [3, 15].

Evaluation failures and fatigue are among the principal causes of injuries. Adequate preparation with the use of proper equipment would reduce the number of injuries in the ski school activities [16]. Older studies shown an incidences of injuries around 1.9–4/1000 runs in professional athletes and up to 80% of them at least one serious injury during their careers. Recently, more accurate data in official competitions have been reported thanks to new methods of data collection and a greater attention [1, 7, 8] (Fig. 6.2).

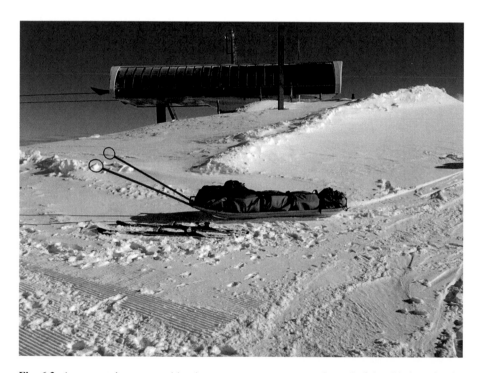

Fig. 6.2 A rescue toboggan used by the rescuers to transport at the end of the ski slope for the injured skier

The number of injuries changed over the years due to several factors. First of all is the evolution of materials and slope-grooming technique. Furthermore, it also changed the type and pattern of injuries. It has gone from a predominance of the tibia and ankle fractures to a prevalence of sprains of the knee [1, 8]. At the beginning of the 1990s, there was a momentous change in the ski equipment: the carving skis. They have different geometry compared with the previous classic skis: they passed from long and slim shape to shorter skis that have a shape with a tight central part and larger extremities. These changes had made skis more maneuverable.

Alpine skiing made its first apparition at the Olympics in 1936, and the first World Cup race was made in 1967 [17].

One athlete in six had a serious injury during each World Cup (WC) season [18]. The International Ski Federation (FIS) had set up the monitoring of accidents in the WC races, both for ski and snowboard, from the 2006 to 2007 season, to have and analyze data over the years. In WC races it happens an injury every 100 runs [19] (Fig. 6.3).

WC alpine skiers had an injury rate of 9.8/1000 runs in the 5-month competitive seasons. It was reported that the downhill discipline had the highest number of injuries every 1000 runs (17.2). Other disciplines follow with 11.0 in super-G, 9.2 in giant slalom, and 4.9 in slalom. Most of the injuries occurred to the knee. Other body districts involved are head, hand, lower leg, lower back, and shoulder. These data were consistent with those of the recreational ski. A difference is found in spine and head injuries that, in recreational ski, often result from falls or collisions with objects along the tracks (trees or lift towers) or other skiers. It was reported that more than half of the injuries, in three consecutive seasons (2006–2009), have forced athletes not to train and participate in competitions for more than a month. Less than a half of the injuries happened in the final part of the races. The injuries

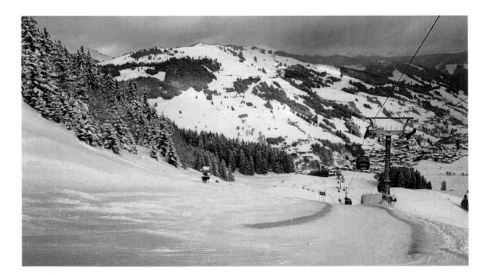

Fig. 6.3 A ski slope of the FIS (International Ski Federation) alpine skiing circuit

occurred mainly in three different situations: while the skier was turning, landing from a jump, both with or without a subsequent fall, and direct consequently to a fall. Gates contributed to the genesis of injuries because, when there is an inappropriate gate contact, they unbalance or disrupt skiing and could lead to an injury directly or indirectly. Skiers could also hooked the gate with the inner ski or their arm [17, 20]. It is very important to have active surveillance systems for injuries. The best way not to lose data is to interview athletes and coaches about the past season. However, this mustn't be the only method [21]. Analysis of the different disciplines must always keep in mind the difference between them. Downhill had the longest course, around 2–4.5 km, that must be run only once with high speed (around 100 km/h maximum), with vertical drop for male up to 1100 m and for female 300 m less [17].

It was found that taking into account the number of injuries per hour of skiing, instead of per runs, there was no difference between DH, GS, and SG. An element that reflects the characteristics of the slopes is the length of the straight sections: up to 45% in DH and only 20% and 7% in SG and GS, respectively. In DH jumps were more frequent with the longest length and airtime [6].

Slalom had two shorter runs with more turns and the maximum vertical drop was 220 m in both sexes. In a recent study, the risk of injury was reported higher in male than in female athletes. This was in contrast with older studies that reported an opposite trend. In addition to this, it was reported that the risk of incidence of knee injuries was comparable between males and females [17]. Still to these days, it remains a topic to be explored with further studies in order to analyze larger and different populations.

Injuries can occur both in competition and in training [22, 23]. The hours of training on the snow of the skiers also include the time of going up to the beginning of the course and wait for the next run. Workouts on the track provide the same exposure to injuries's risks as in the race. With modern techniques of training, a lot of time is dedicated to the preparation of the snow, especially during the summer season. Then in these situations, which mostly happen in the gym, the accidents possible are common to all types of sports. In children and adolescents, all risk factors involved in adults are present (fatigue, experience, etc.), with the addition of some age-related factors: musculoskeletal immaturity, age, and equipment. Incommensurable bone growth and skeletal development were involved in around 15% of injuries in children. Muscular weakness, fatigue, and musculoskeletal imbalances were other elements that contribute to the genesis of injuries. Modern equipment, and in particular boots, were made of stiff plastic and dress a great part of the tibia, stopping on the proximal third. These characteristics focus the pivot's force on the tibial shaft and, considering lower bone strength and tibia's sections of children, they result in a weak point. Twisting forces, or sprain, could lead to fractures more easily than adults. It has been reported in literature that up to 50% of accidents occur in inexperienced children on the first day of ski practice and education. Another critical period is the beginning of the winter season where many will approach skiing without proper physical preparation. It is reported that the number of accidents in children followed a bimodal trend. First peak was caused by young inexperienced skiers with limited skills in movement. Second peak was represented by experienced skiers who push themselves beyond their limits [2]. In our series (data from FISI—Italian Winter Sports Federation), injuries usually involved in order of frequency: 52% knee, 9% ankle, 9% head, 8% torso, 6% shoulder, 6% lower leg, 4% miscellaneous, 3% hand, and 3% thigh.

6.1 Lower Limbs

More than half of injuries to the lower limbs, in the Alpine Ski World Cup, involved the knee and almost all occur while the athlete is still skiing or before the fall. Fractures and bruises represent mostly of the other half of injuries [20]. The ski binding release was a key point in the genesis or protection of the lower limb injuries [8]. Injuries involving the lower limbs in children are three times more frequent than in adults. Fractures in children skiers under 10 years old are nine times more frequent than in adults. Up to one-fifth of these injuries were reported to be femoral fractures, due to collisions, high speed, and falls. In literature, it was reported that the knee is the anatomical region subjected to the higher number of trauma, also in young people. Knee sprains mainly lead to anterior cruciate ligament (ACL) and the medial collateral ligament (MCL) injuries, like in adults. It's not uncommon to find in these young population ligament injury associated with fracture. Distal femoral fracture involving the growth plate (Salter-Harris) was reported to be frequent. In children and adolescents, tibia and fibula fractures had also a high frequency. Tibia fractures of the middle distal third usually had an isolated spiral or multifragmentary pattern. Tibial plateau fractures, associated or not with ligament injuries, were result of knee sprain and their incidence was rising, mainly as a fracture of intercondylar spine [2]. In our series (data from FISI—Italian Winter Sports Federation), injuries of the lower limb usually involved in order of frequency: 72% knee, 12% ankle, 9% lower leg, 4% thigh, and 2% hip. If the knee was involved, we have this frequency of type of trauma: 66% sprains, 16% fractures, 10% contusions, 3% wounds, 3% chondral lesions, and 2% dislocations.

6.1.1 Knee Sprain

A knee sprain usually caused an ACL or a medial collateral ligament (MCL) injury [24]. Also meniscal lesions and bone marrow edema were often found after a knee sprain. The MCL injuries were of low grade (I and II) in most cases and need a non-operative treatment [24].

We have witnessed the evolution of equipment in recent decades, but despite the latest innovations, in recent years, the number of ACL injuries is roughly the same. The ACL injury mechanism is due to the slip and catch skiing technique, needed with the new skis, which lead athletes' knee to flexion and internal rotation. International Ski Federation (FIS) in 2012 published new rules to try to decrease these types of injuries, with the reduction of turning radius and aggressiveness of the skies [8]. An element which acts as a cause, or way, of knee's injury is the ski binding release. It has been reported that skis act as a lever during the fall, or the torsional movement, and lead to a knee injury before the binding release or because the release never happens [17, 20].

6.1.1.1   Mechanisms of Anterior Cruciate Ligament Injury

There are specific mechanisms of ACL injury in skiers. In recreational skiers, the phantom foot is the most common. The skier was imbalanced backward with the omolateral knee and hip flexed. The hip is under the level of the knee. In this position, the ski could act as a lever, if it takes the direction to the other leg and creates a constrained internal rotation of the flexed knee that could lead to ACL injury [24, 25] (Fig. 6.4a).

The second mechanism is the boot-induced anterior drawer (BIAD). It happens when the skier is landing on the ski tail from a jump with an imbalance backward and the knees almost extended. On landing, loads are transmitted from ski to the binding and then to the boot. The tibia undergoes to a forward shift (anterior drawer) that could have enough energy to injure the ACL. Other elements could be involved in the BIAD mechanism, although they certainly are more involved in the World Cup skiers/elite. One is a tibio-femoral vertical compression force that could add stress to the ACL. Another is a lower activation of the knee flexors than the extensors (hamstrings and quadriceps). Even a strong contraction of the quadriceps to get back into the correct position and/or hyperflexion of the knee when landing from a jump have been considered in the literature as factors of additional stress to the ACL in addition to the BIAD [24, 25] (Fig. 6.4b). The third ACL injury mechanism in recreational alpine skiers is the classic *valgus-external rotation*. It occurs when there is a forward fall and at the same time the tip of the ski hits the snow. Then the ski could do an external twist and leads the knee in external rotation with the tibia in valgus. In this type of mechanism, the MCL is involved a lot of times and it can be the only injured ligament. It has been supposed that the diffusion of carving skis

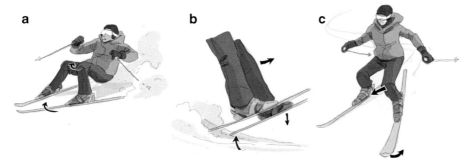

Fig. 6.4 Mechanisms of anterior cruciate ligament injury in recreational skiers. (**a**) Phantom foot. (**b**) Boot-induced anterior drawer. (**c**) Valgus-external rotation (Illustrations by Alberto Madrigal)

had led to an increase of valgus-external rotation injury due to the characteristics of the ski and the ski technique [24, 25] (Fig. 6.4c).

In World Cup alpine skiing, a detailed analysis of ACL injury mechanisms was made by analyzing videos of athletes' injuries: three typical ACL injury mechanisms in professional alpine skiers were defined. The pattern, set, and background are different between recreational and elite skiers. The first element which will lead to the injury, regardless of the mechanism, is almost always a technical error, or tactical, of the skier which leads to an imbalance, forward or backward [26].

The slip-catch mechanism was based on a loss of balance while the skier was facing a turn. The outer ski should take the curve's tangential trajectory and consequently went away from the body's center of mass. When the skier tried to extend the leg (Fig. 6.5a) to recover the support and the balance with the outer ski,

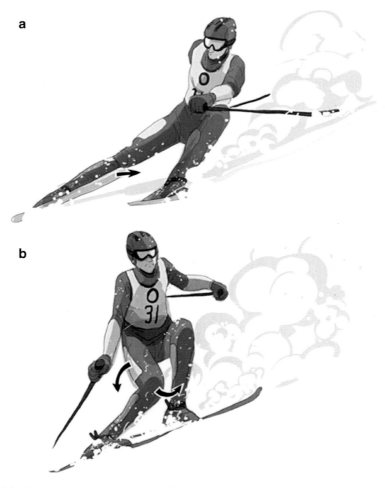

Fig. 6.5 Two consecutive phases of the slip-catch mechanism of anterior cruciate ligament injury in elite skiers. **a**) The skier's movement that predisposes to the injury's mechanism **b**) The resulting movement that could causes knee injuries (Illustrations by Alberto Madrigal)

the sudden grip with snow could lead to injury: the knee was twisted in an internal rotation, flexion, and valgus movement that puts a strain on the ligaments (Fig. 6.5b). A biomechanical study also highlighted the importance of knee's compression in the genesis of the injury [26, 27].

The dynamic snowplow mechanism started with a ski erroneously unloaded by body weight that, driven by the snow, went away from the center of the body. In this unbalanced situation, the loaded ski oscillated from the inner to the outer edge leading to a knee sprain with an internal rotation and/or valgus movement (Fig. 6.6a). The landing back-weighted mechanism is generated by a technical error in the jump that takes the skier to land with the weight backward on the tail of the skis with a large clap angle (the angle formed by the axis of the ski and the axis parallel to the ground) and the knee extended. When the ski rotated to be parallel to the ground, using the tail of the ski as pivot, the knee was forced to suffer a femorotibial compression and an anterior drawer. The skier, in the while, tried to recover and fell backward. Some of the concepts of this mechanism are shared with the BIAD

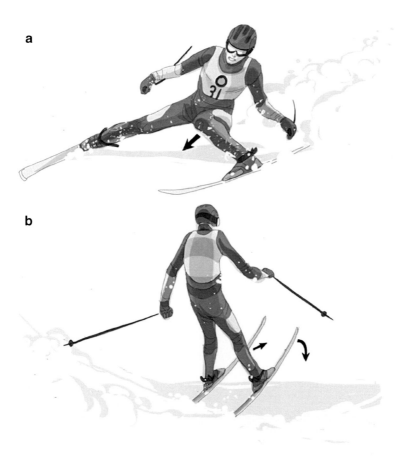

Fig. 6.6 Mechanisms of anterior cruciate ligament injury in elite skiers. (**a**) Dynamic snowplow. (**b**) Landing back-weighted (Illustrations by Alberto Madrigal)

mechanism of the recreational skiers, but it is described separately as landing back-weighted because it occurs in the presence of much higher and more forces that could stress the ACL. These forces are involved, as described before, even when the elite skier attempts to recover from the falling-back position with the muscle contraction and when the tibio-femoral vertical compression force acts on the knee and on the ACL, as a result of the landing [26] (Fig. 6.6b).

A high momentum of forces through the ACL, which could lead to an injury, was reported to be there if the athletes, in a land from a jump, had hip flexed and knee extended or was in an asymmetric position. Among all the variables, the back position in a jump landing was the most predictive element in ACL injuries [28].

Slip-catch is reported to be the main ACL injury's mechanism in WC. However, in our series (data from FISI—Italian Winter Sports Federation), the most common mechanism remains the valgus-external rotation. In our experiences, the introduction of side-cut skis had increased the number of ACL injuries with valgus-external rotation mechanism and, on the other hand, the new skis with increased side-cut radius have reduced this trend.

Meniscal tears associated with ACL injuries were reported to be around a quarter or half of the ACL tears. This rate in skiers was lower than the one reported by other sports. If ACL and MCL are injured, the lateral meniscus tear is very common. Lateral collateral ligament and posterior cruciate ligament (PCL) injuries were rare. They used to be present in knee dislocations in which you always had to suspect a vascular and/or nerve injury [24].

6.1.1.2 Imaging

Magnetic resonance imaging (MRI) is the gold standard radiological exam to evaluate capsular ligament injuries in knee sprains after performing X-rays in case of an acute trauma [24] (Fig. 6.7). X-rays show fractures and/or indirect signs of other injuries. MRI also shows the extension of the bone marrow edema.

Knee sprain can also lead to fractures due to the traction made by ligaments on their bone insertions. Pathognomonic of a varus trauma is the Segond fracture.

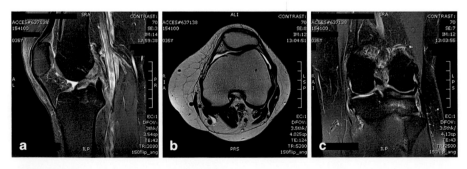

Fig. 6.7 Magnetic resonance imaging (MRI) of a knee with an anterior cruciate ligament lesion. (**a**) Sagittal view. (**b**) Axial view. (**c**) Coronal view

X-rays show the avulsion of the tibial lateral condyle at the lateral collateral ligament insertion [29].

6.1.1.3 Management

After a sprain, the knee can become very swollen and then increase the pain and limit the movements. In selected cases, it may be appropriate to perform an arthrocentesis to reduce the symptoms. The knee joint aspiration has to be performed, in our experience, only if the knee is very swollen and symptomatic. In the case of injury of anterior cruciate ligament, usually, blood is aspirated. Also in articular knee fractures, it can be present in hemarthrosis. In the first days, the knee should be treated with ice and rest. Radiological diagnosis and physical examination let to decide the therapeutic course for the athlete. Fractures require immobilization and weight unloading on the injured lower limb. A knee sprain without fractures allows to walk when swelling and pain will be reduced [30, 31]. In high-level athletes, if the knee allows and/or if there are associated injuries, reconstructive surgery of the ligaments can also be done the same day or the day after the trauma, always in accordance with the athlete.In isolated lesions of ACL, we used to reconstruct the ligament with autologous and ipsilateral hamstrings. We prefer hamstring to patellar tendon to avoid weakening of the extensor apparatus and to avoid important patellar tendinopathy, which in our series, in some cases in the past, took place after the surgery. In skiing, the eccentric quadriceps strength is crucial, so we prefer not to weaken it, and preserve it, when it's possible (Fig. 6.8). In the presence of

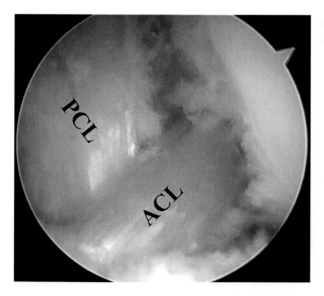

Fig. 6.8 Arthroscopic view of a reconstructed anterior cruciate ligament (ACL) with hamstrings and of the posterior cruciate ligament (PCL)

multi-ligament injuries and/or of particular associated lesions, the allograft becomes, in our experience, the graft of first choice in ligaments' reconstruction surgery.

6.1.1.4   Physiotherapy

In most cases, physiotherapy should be started immediately, both awaiting the surgery and immediately after it. It must respect the inflammatory knee condition, especially when you are very close at the time of the trauma and/or surgery, and its response to physiotherapy exercises. ACL injuries were common and consequently there were skiers who returned to sports after an ACL reconstruction. A study has shown that in skiers with an ACL reconstruction, there was an asymmetry between lower limbs both functional and muscles' mass compared to skiers who have not undergone any surgery [32].

It has also been reported a significant loss of maximum quadriceps and hamstring strength in the operated limb, compared to the contralateral and with not injured athletes [33].

The introduction of exercises aimed at proprioception, as early as possible, improved the muscles' strength and some functional outcome better and before (up to 2 months in advance) than athletes who have faced a rehabilitation without these elements [34].

Athletes must therefore do a physiotherapy work, for return to sport after ACL reconstruction, focused on muscles' strengthening and on functional recovery. This program should be done even after the resumption of sporting gesture. Proprioception and core stability are two key concepts to keep in mind the return to sport after knee's ligament reconstruction surgery. In addition to this, we must never forget the respect of biological healing time: we can't accelerate beyond biology. At 4–4.5 months, if there is a good proprioception and neuromuscular recovery, controlled by field tests, the athlete can start skiing in free field at proprioceptive purpose, for a reathletization sports specific. A low level of proprioception of the knee can be improved with kinesiology tape (KT). People with injuries or after surgery can get benefits, in the first period, from the application of KT, but it mustn't be a routine [35].

The proprioception of the knee is not affected by use of knee supports [36].

In young skiers, a risk factor to ACL injury is the core strength deficits. This should be a target of trainings [37].

6.1.2   Fractures

With the introduction of stiff ski boots, fractures of the tibia and ankle sprain were decreased significantly. The ski binding release systems helped to decrease the incidence of spiral tibial shaft fractures but they are still present in cases of malfunctioning of bindings (boot top fractures) [24]. Young or novice skiers were reported to have a lot of tibial diaphysis fractures. Expert skiers used to have a fracture pattern that includes the whole tibia. The use of snowblades increased the risk of a lower limb fractures. A problem in the binding release is the most common cause. The mechanism that results more is rotational trauma [38].

However, we mustn't forget that since bindings were introduced they have significantly reduced the incidence of tibial fractures [12].

The introduction of the carving ski started to increase the number of complex proximal tibia fractures that before were uncommon [39].

The same forces transmitted to the knee, which increased the number of knee sprains, could cause fractures of the tibial plateau [24].

In a prospective study of more than 10 years, a reduction of 89% of the number of tibia fractures in adults and a simultaneous increase of the ACL injuries 280% were reported. The average number of injuries has dropped over time for both adults and children and adolescents [40].

X-rays in case of suspected fracture must always be done. A computed tomography (CT) is required to evaluate the intra-articular involvement in the case of tibial plateau fractures or shaft long fractures [24].

Fractures of the lower limb properly treated allowed to return to previous competitive levels [41, 42]. It is a high-speed sport; therefore, although with a lower incidence, vertebral and femoral fractures were reported in literature and in our series. Despite the protections are improving and evolving, fractures are always present, even because athletes fall on slopes even more harsh and more energy is involved in injuries. Non-displaced fractures could be treated conservatively. Unstable or displaced fractures, especially if are intra-articular, require a surgical treatment in most cases. In the treatment of fractures that require surgical intervention, the choice of the implants must also take into account the patient-athlete and its functional requirements. In the skiers we prefer to use, when the fracture's pattern allows it, implants that will not interfere with the sport later: in our experience, when it's possible, we prefer and we use intramedullary nails rather than plates.

This is because a tibial plate is very superficial and it can give problems and discomfort with continued use of the boot and its repeated pressure on the skin over the plate.

6.1.3 Cartilage Lesions

Joints' cartilage could undergo disease processes often with unknown etiology, such as osteochondritis dissecans, or with traumatic injuries as a result of sprain or direct trauma. Treatments for cartilage lesions were very delicate and difficult but with the correct indications could get excellent results. Skiers with cartilage defects were treated with microfractures with good results, and they reached the final goal to return to race in competitions. Advanced treatments with AMIC technique may be the right weapon to treat osteochondritis dissecans or more complex cartilage injuries also in joints different from the knee, like the ankle [43, 44]. Cartilage injuries are difficult to treat and it is more difficult to get good results in the long term.

Cartilage injuries are not only caused by traumatic injuries but can also be caused by overuse injuries. In skiing both of these etiological factors are present: it is an arduous sport and, as we have seen, joints could have continuous traumas.

6.2 Upper Limbs

In World Cup races, injuries of the back and torso were caused mainly in speed disciplines due to a hit on the snow surface or on the safety net in a fall. Fractures of the lumbar spine and contusion to the lower back and ribs were reported. On the other side, injuries of the upper limb were reported both in technical and speed disciplines. The most frequent injuries of the upper limb were, first of all, the fractures of the bones, followed by acromioclavicular and glenohumeral joint dislocations [20]. Therefore, injuries to the upper limbs mostly occur from falls [7].

Shoulder injuries were underestimated because skiers with this type of injury usually preferred go to their local medical specialist rather than to ski emergency room. In some types of injuries, only a quarter of the patients seek for an immediate medical consultation. Therefore in literature shoulder injuries were reported to be only 4–11% of all alpine skiing injuries [45]. In recent years, even though injuries are declining in incidence, fractures of the humerus and clavicle, at the same time, have a reverse trend. The latter indeed happen more often, and their mechanism is usually a direct trauma on the shoulder [45]. In recent years, we have seen, both in literature than in our series, an increase of the upper limb and hand fractures, particularly of the metacarpals. This is due to the evolution of skiing techniques: the arm and hand have become a third support on the snow to compensate for the tilt of the body and its imbalance. Despite the protections, the presence of an increasingly hard snow has encouraged this increase. In the top level athletes, some upper limb fractures treated surgically with good osteosynthesis and with appropriate protections allow an early return to sports, although with some risk factors. An increasing rate of injuries of the upper limb in children was reported; this is probably due to the increase in the number of cases of thumb impairment. But most of the injuries involved the shoulder and were clavicle fractures, acromioclavicular dislocations, and humeral fractures. Salter-Harris type I and II fractures of the proximal phalanx were more common in children under 13 years old. Adolescents usually had metacarpophalangeal sprains and injuries of the ulnar collateral ligament (partial or complete rupture, the skier's thumb) often associated with bony avulsion (Stener lesion) [2]. Skiers had less frequently abdominal injuries compared to snowboarders, in particular of the spleen, and consequently the need of surgery [7]. In our series (data from FISI—Italian Winter Sports Federation), injuries of the upper limb were in order of frequency: 37% fractures, 22% dislocations, 22% contusions, 8% wounds, 8% sprains, and 3% miscellaneous. These upper limb injuries, in our series, involved in order of frequency: 51% shoulder, 28% wrist/hand, 9% elbow, 6% arm, and 6% forearm.

6.2.1 Shoulder Injuries

A direct fall on the shoulder, or arm, can cause injuries, like in the other sports. In addition to this, in alpine ski there is a specific sport-related mechanism of shoulder injury, the pole planting. It happens when the pole is sticked in the snow or catched by something on the slope which leads to an anterior dislocation of the glenohumeral joint [20].

In alpine skiing, shoulder injuries were reported to have a rate of 0.2–0.5 injuries/1000 skier-days [24].

Among shoulder injuries in this sport, in order of frequency, rotator cuff strains, glenohumeral dislocations and subluxations, acromionclavear dislocations, and clavicle fractures were reported. The shoulder could be injured by specific mechanisms: a direct hit on it, an eccentric strength with the arm opposite to abduction movement or an axial load generated on an extended arm. Certainly, classic traumas mustn't be forgotten, such as movements forced in extrarotation by the ski poles planted in the snow and collisions with objects or other people. Wrist straps of the ski poles connected with skier's wrist could pull the upper limb if they remained planted in the snow [45]. The humeral fractures in recreational skiers were reported in literature to have a lower incidence compared to snowboarders. An incidence of humeral fractures in recreational skiers of 0.041/1000 skiers-day was calculated [46].

Adolescents had a lower risk of shoulder injuries than children and adults. Children used to have a fracture when the shoulder is involved and adults used to have dislocations [12]. Shoulder dislocations must be treated as soon as possible in a protected environment with X-rays before and after reduction (Fig. 6.9). Vascular and nerve complications are the most dangerous in this injuries and have always to be taken into account in the management of patients. The pole, by acting as leverage in certain situations, could suddenly load forces on the shoulder causing more easily

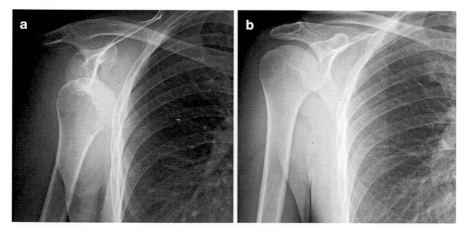

Fig. 6.9 Shoulder dislocation. (**a**) X-rays before reduction. (**b**) X-rays after reduction

dislocation. The lower the age at the time of the first episode, the higher the probability to have a recurrence. In a patient, more than 40 years old, with a shoulder dislocation, we have to suspect an injury of the rotator cuff. The rate of shoulder injuries in children remains high despite security measures that are used more and more [45].

Clavicle fractures used to result from a direct fall on the acromion. Most of the fractures involved the middle third and if not a lot of displaced could be treated conservatively [24]. Medial and lateral third fractures were less common.

Fractures of the medial third must be studied carefully because they could cause secondary vascular injury if they were displaced posteriorly [47]. The treatment of clavicle fractures can be nonoperative with the figure-of-eight bandage, especially in the middle third fractures non-displaced, or operative with a plate and screws or intramedullary fixation [31]. In our vision, to let the athletes return as quickly as possible to ski again and make them lose less time as possible, we prefer a surgical approach always informing athletes about all the risks, benefits, and alternatives.

6.2.2   Thumb and Hand Injuries

The typical hand trauma is due to a fall with the ski pole held in the hand that cause a traumatic hyperabduction and extension of the first metacarpophalangeal joint (MCP), called skier's thumb. This resulted in a sprain of the thumb ulnar collateral ligament (UCL) [20, 45].

An important element that supports the UCL injuries in skiers is the high fall's kinetic energy down the slope which is transmitted into a valgus movement of the MCP.

In addition to this, it was reported that the pole acts as a lever on the MCP which causes Stener lesions to happen easily. The Stener lesion happens when the ulnar expansion of the dorsal aponeurosis moved between the injured ligament and its insertion on the proximal phalanx. This situation causes a palpable swelling which is painful at the site of the ligament balled up. It was suggested that the use of pole straps could increase this type of injuries. The first indirect sign of UCL injury is the evidence at the X-ray of an avulsion fracture of the base of the proximal phalanx of the thumb. If there aren't bone fractures, the symptoms related with the physical examination and magnetic resonance imaging (MRI) or ultrasound (US) make the diagnosis [24].

In a wrist injury must always suspect a fracture of the scaphoid. A suspected scaphoid fracture, in the absence of evidence of fracture on X-rays, must always investigated with MRI.

6.3   Fatal Injuries

The National Ski Areas Association (NSAA) annually reported data from all the US ski areas. In the last 10 years, an average of 38 deaths occurred every season among skiers and snowboarders.

In the 2015/2016 season, they have 52.8 million skier/snowboarder days with 39 fatalities. Among these fatalities, 7 were snowboarders and 31 were skiers (NSAA didn't know equipment data about one of these). Male gender was the most frequent with 79.5% and the helmet was worn at the time of the accident by 23 people.

NSAA reported that four-fifths of all skiers in the United States wore helmets in the last season. The rate of fatality in the 2015/2016 season was 0.74/1 million skiers/snowboarders. We are faced with a minimal increase of this data but remains in the average for the last few years. These numbers are much lower than those of other causes of death, but must not be underestimated. The data reported from the NSAA did not include deaths caused by underlying medical conditions or deaths of ski area's employees. The fatalities reported were those that happened in the ski area's boundaries and did not include those in the backcountry (off-piste or out of area) [48]. The most common cause of traumatic fatalities is a clash with an object on the slope, such as another skier or snowboard, trees, or poles. Head injuries, isolated or in association with other injuries, were frequent cause of death [49]. The deaths of World Cup athletes, especially in recent times, are very rare.

In recent history, we remember Ulrike Maier who died in 1994 in Garmisch (due to a head/neck trauma against a snowbank), Gernot Reinstadler who died in Wengen in 1991 (as a result of injuries sustained in the fall), and Régine Cavagnoud who died in 2001 (as a result of a high-speed collision during training in Pitztal). In the same years, there have been incidents that have not led to the death but have led to disabling outcomes. In 1995, Thomas Fogdoe got a motor disability of the lower limbs as a result of a training accident. In 2001, in Val d'Isere, Silvano Beltrametti had the same fate because of a high-energy fall that made him break through the security nets. In 2008, in Kvitfjell, Matthias Lanzinger underwent the amputation of a lower leg as a result of injuries sustained in a crash. The helmet is an important safety device that must always be worn while skiing.

In the literature, there is a lack of information concerning the fatal injuries in the general population and particularly in children. A death certificate-based surveillance system reported an average of one child death per year in a period of 21 years before the spread of the use of the helmet on the slopes: the number of fatal injuries reported in children was 14% of the total, including adults. The most common cause of death in skiers from 7 to 17 years old was reported to be traumatic brain injury [2, 50].

References

1. Koehle MS, Lloyd-Smith R, Taunton JE (2002) Alpine ski injuries and their prevention. Sports Med 32(12):785–793
2. Meyers MC, Laurent CM Jr, Higgins RW, Skelly WA (2007) Downhill ski injuries in children and adolescents. Sports Med 37(6):485–499
3. Coury T, Napoli AM, Wilson M, Daniels J, Murray R, Milzman D (2013) Injury patterns in recreational alpine skiing and snowboarding at a mountainside clinic. Wilderness Environ Med 24(4):417–421

4. Ruedl G, Kopp M, Sommersacher R, Woldrich T, Burtscher M (2013) Factors associated with injuries occurred on slope intersections and in snow parks compared to on-slope injuries. Accid Anal Prev 50:1221–1225
5. Flørenes TW, Nordsletten L, Heir S, Bahr R (2012) Injuries among World Cup ski and snowboard athletes. Scand J Med Sci Sports 22(1):58–66
6. Gilgien M, Spörri J, Kröll J, Crivelli P, Müller E (2014) Mechanics of turning and jumping and skier speed are associated with injury risk in men's World Cup alpine skiing: a comparison between the competition disciplines. Br J Sports Med 48(9):742–747
7. McBeth PB, Ball CG, Mulloy RH, Kirkpatrick AW (2009) Alpine ski and snowboarding traumatic injuries: incidence, injury patterns, and risk factors for 10 years. Am J Surg 197(5):560–563. discussion 563–4
8. Stenroos AJ, Handolin LE (2014) Alpine skiing injuries in Finland – a two-year retrospective study based on a questionnaire among ski racers. BMC Sports Sci Med Rehabil 6(1):9
9. Ruedl G, Kopp M, Burtscher M, Bauer R, Benedetto K (2013) Ursachen und Einflussfaktoren von Personenkollisionen auf der Skipiste – causes and factors associated with collisions on ski slopes. Sportverletz Sportschaden 27(2):100–104
10. Philippe M, Ruedl G, Feltus G, Woldrich T, Burtscher M (2014) How frequent and why are skiers and snowboarders falling? Sportverletz Sportschaden 28(4):188–192
11. Rust DA, Gilmore CJ, Treme G (2013) Injury patterns at a large Western United States ski resort with and without snowboarders: the Taos experience. Am J Sports Med 41(3):652–656
12. Sulheim S, Holme I, Rødven A, Ekeland A, Bahr R (2011) Risk factors for injuries in alpine skiing, telemark skiing and snowboarding—case-control study. Br J Sports Med 45(16):1303–1309
13. Bere T, Flørenes TW, Nordsletten L, Bahr R (2014) Sex differences in the risk of injury in World Cup alpine skiers: a 6-year cohort study. Br J Sports Med 48(1):36–40
14. Heir S, Krosshaug T, Rødven A Ekeland A (2002) Injuries in alpine skiing related to age groups. Paper presented at the 10th ESSKA Congress
15. Westin M, Alricsson M, Werner S (2012) Injury profile of competitive alpine skiers: a five-year cohort study. Knee Surg Sports Traumatol Arthrosc 20(6):1175–1181
16. Greier K (2011) Skiing injuries in school sport and possibilities to prevent them. Sportverletz Sportschaden 25(4):216–221
17. Flørenes TW, Bere T, Nordsletten L, Heir S, Bahr R (2009) Injuries among male and female World Cup alpine skiers. Br J Sports Med 43(13):973–978
18. Gilgien M, Crivelli P, Spörri J, Kröll J, Müller E (2015) Characterization of course and terrain and their effect on skier speed in World Cup alpine ski racing. PLoS One 10(3):e0118119
19. Bere T, Bahr R (2014) Injury prevention advances in alpine ski racing: harnessing collaboration with the International Ski Federation (FIS), long-term surveillance and digital technology to benefit athletes. Br J Sports Med 48(9):738
20. Bere T, Flørenes TW, Krosshaug T, Haugen P, Svandal I, Nordsletten L, Bahr R (2014) A systematic video analysis of 69 injury cases in World Cup alpine skiing. Scand J Med Sci Sports 24(4):667–677
21. Flørenes TW, Nordsletten L, Heir S, Bahr R (2011) Recording injuries among World Cup skiers and snowboarders: a methodological study. Scand J Med Sci Sports 21(2):196–205
22. Ruedl G, Schobersberger W, Pocecco E, Blank C, Engebretsen L, Soligard T, Steffen K, Kopp M, Burtscher M (2012) Sport injuries and illnesses during the first Winter Youth Olympic Games 2012 in Innsbruck. Austria Br J Sports Med 46(15):1030–1037
23. Ruedl G, Schnitzer M, Kirschner W, Spiegel R, Platzgummer H, Kopp M, Burtscher M, Pocecco E (2016) Sport injuries and illnesses during the 2015 Winter European Youth Olympic Festival. Br J Sports Med 50(10):631–636
24. Deady LH, Salonen D (2010) Skiing and snowboarding injuries: a review with a focus on mechanism of injury. Radiol Clin N Am 48(6):1113–1124
25. Shea KG, Archibald-Seiffer N, Murdock E, Grimm NL, Jacobs JC Jr, Willick S, Van Houten H (2014) Knee injuries in downhill skiers: a 6-year survey study. Orthop J Sports Med 2(1):2325967113519741

26. Bere T, Flørenes TW, Krosshaug T, Nordsletten L, Bahr R (2011) Events leading to anterior cruciate ligament injury in World Cup Alpine Skiing: a systematic video analysis of 20 cases. Br J Sports Med 45(16):1294–1302

27. Bere T, Mok KM, Koga H, Krosshaug T, Nordsletten L, Bahr R (2013) Kinematics of anterior cruciate ligament ruptures in World Cup alpine skiing: 2 case reports of the slip-catch mechanism. Am J Sports Med 41(5):1067–1073

28. Heinrich D, van den Bogert AJ, Nachbauer W (2014) Relationship between jump landing kinematics and peak ACL force during a jump in downhill skiing: a simulation study. Scand J Med Sci Sports 24(3):e180–e187

29. Abdalla FH, Tehranzadeh J, Horton JA (1982) Avulsion of lateral tibial condyle in skiing. Am J Sports Med 10(6):368–370

30. Brukner P (2012) Brukner and Khan's clinical sports medicine. McGraw-Hill, North Ryde

31. Canale ST, Beaty JH (2012) Campbell's operative orthopaedics, XI edn. Elsevier Health Sciences, Philadelphia, PA

32. Jordan MJ, Aagaard P, Herzog W (2015) Lower limb asymmetry in mechanical muscle function: a comparison between ski racers with and without ACL reconstruction. Scand J Med Sci Sports 25(3):e301–e309

33. Jordan MJ, Aagaard P, Herzog W (2015) Rapid hamstrings/quadriceps strength in ACL-reconstructed elite Alpine ski racers. Med Sci Sports Exerc 47(1):109–119

34. Sidorenko EV, Preobrazhenskiĭ VIu, Vnukov DV, Preobrazhenskaia MV (2013) [Peculiarities of early rehabilitation of mountain ski athletes after plastic reconstruction of anterior cruciate ligament]. Vopr Kurortol Fizioter Lech Fiz Kult. Jul-Aug;(4):35–38.

35. Hosp S, Bottoni G, Heinrich D, Kofler P, Hasler M, Nachbauer W (2015) A pilot study of the effect of kinesiology tape on knee proprioception after physical activity in healthy women. J Sci Med Sport 18(6):709–713

36. Bottoni G, Herten A, Kofler P, Hasler M, Nachbauer W (2013) The effect of knee brace and knee sleeve on the proprioception of the knee in young non-professional healthy sportsmen. Knee 20(6):490–492

37. Raschner C, Platzer HP, Patterson C, Werner I, Huber R, Hildebrandt C (2012) The relationship between ACL injuries and physical fitness in young competitive ski racers: a 10-year longitudinal study. Br J Sports Med 46(15):1065–1071

38. Bürkner A, Simmen HP (2008) Fractures of the lower extremity in skiing - the influence of ski boots and injury pattern. Sportverletz Sportschaden 22(4):207–212

39. Pätzold R, Spiegl U, Wurster M, Augat P, Gutsfeld P, Gonschorek O, Bühren V (2013) Proximal tibial fractures sustained during alpine skiing – incidence and risk factors. Sportverletz Sportschaden 27(4):207–211

40. Deibert MC, Aronsson DD, Johnson RJ, Ettlinger CF, Shealy JE (1998) Skiing injuries in children, adolescents, and adults. J Bone Joint Surg Am 80(1):25–32

41. Mückley T, Kruis C, Schütz T, Brucker P, Bühren V (2004) Fractures of the lower leg in professional skiers. Sportverletz Sportschaden 18(1):22–27

42. Pavić R (2012) Multifragmentary distal crural fracture ski injury in an athlete: a case report. Coll Antropol 36(4):1471–1474

43. Hotfiel T, Engelhardt M (2015) Osteochondritis dissecans of the talus with hindfoot malalignment—autologous matrix-induced chondrogenesis with lateral calcaneal distraction osteotomy in an internationally successful young female ski racer. Sportverletz Sportschaden 29(2):118–121

44. Steadman JR, Hanson CM, Briggs KK, Matheny LM, James EW, Guillet A (2014) Outcomes after knee microfracture of chondral defects in alpine ski racers. J Knee Surg 27(5):407–410

45. McCall D, Safran MR (2009) Injuries about the shoulder in skiing and snowboarding. Br J Sports Med 43(13):987–992

46. Bissell BT, Johnson RJ, Shafritz AB, Chase DC, Ettlinger CF (2008) Epidemiology and risk factors of humerus fractures among skiers and snowboarders. Am J Sports Med 36(10):1880–1888

47. di Mento L, Staletti L, Cavanna M, Mocchi M, Berlusconi M (2015) Posterior sternoclavicular joint dislocation with brachiocephalic vein injury: a case report. Injury 46(Suppl 7):S8–10
48. National Ski Areas Association (2016) Facts about skiing/snowboarding safety. NSAA Online publications. http://www.nsaa.org
49. Shealy J, Johnson R, Ettlinger C (2006) On piste fatalities in recreational snow sports in the US. Skiing trauma and safety 16th volume. ASTM STP 1474:27–34
50. Xiang H, Stallones L, Smith GA (2004) Downhill skiing injury fatalities among children. Inj Prev 10(2):99–102

Chapter 7
Overuse Injuries in Alpine Skiers

Gabriele Thiébat, Andrea Panzeri, Paolo Capitani, and Herbert Schoenhuber

Abstract Overuse injuries are common in all sports and also in Alpine Ski. In this discipline they can happen in the dry-land trainings or on the snow, both in races or training. The first ones are common to all the sports, while on the snow are uniques for the Winter Sports. New training techniques have increased the workload of some anatomical districts, going to increase the incidence of overuse injuries.

There are few reports in the literature on overuse injuries in skiing. The exact incidence is often not known, because many studies are more focused on acute traumas. New studies are definitely needed to better define this group of injuries that have a big negative impact on the performance of athletes.

7.1 Low Back Pain

The anatomic region of the most common overuse injuries in Alpine ski is the back. The incidence of lower back pain in athletes who practice this sport is significantly higher than the normal population. Recurring and immoderate back loads were gradually adding up over the years, becoming a mechanical cause of overuse injuries of the back. Another key element was the technical gestures performed in the sport that increase stress on the discs. It was reported during carved ski turns loads on the back achieve up to 2.89 times the body weight. This latter element associated with the torsion of the torso and bending needed for skiing was the starter element of back pathologies. Also the shapes of the slopes could affect these loads. A recent study reports that in slalom (SL) the back benefits from a reduction of the loads if the gate offset was increased [1].

G. Thiébat (✉) • A. Panzeri • P. Capitani • H. Schoenhuber
Sport Traumatology Centre, IRCCS Istituto Ortopedico Galeazzi,
Via Riccardo Galeazzi 4, 20161 Milano, Italy
e-mail: gthiebat@gmail.com; paolocapitani.dr@gmail.com

© Springer International Publishing AG 2018   77
H. Schoenhuber et al. (eds.), *Alpine Skiing Injuries*, Sports and Traumatology,
https://doi.org/10.1007/978-3-319-61355-0_7

When an unexpected factor arises while the athletes are skiing, such as a trauma, an injury, or an error in the skiing technique, the loads on the back can increase significantly over the data previously reported.

The skiing techniques should focus on the control and reduction of the torsion and lateral and frontal bending because they increased the load on the spinal disc [1].

Especially in the last two seasons, we have seen, among our athletes, an increased incidence of low back pain, also for the evolution of the technical materials used. Our athletes reported that more and more force and energy are needed to control the ski equipment. In relation to these data and to other reports, the International Ski Federation (FIS) from the next season (2017/2018) wants to further modify the side-cut radius to help reduce the incidence of low back pain and other injuries. Today in high-level skiers, low back pain is becoming one of the most frequent injuries, after knee sprains.

7.1.1 Diagnosis and Management

A precise diagnosis of the cause of back pain isn't easy to make. Only in a tenth of patients it could be possible to identify a specific cause. Even without an anatomical or structural diagnosis, it is possible to manage the low back pain.

It is often a combination of factors that cause low back pain. A degenerative disc disease may be associated with facet joint syndromes that together give the set of symptoms.

Vertebral fractures of the lumbar spine can be caused by direct trauma, compressive or torsional. These fractures can involve all the vertebral anatomical parts.

The clinical presentation of a patient with a nerve root compression is usually pathognomonic. Symptoms and sensory or motor alterations, irradiated to one or both lower limbs, help to identify the level of the lesion. A low back pain can be associated or not. Spinal canal stenosis is very uncommon in young and adult, up to 50 years, skiers.

Stress fractures and spondylolysis in ski athletes may occur due to the continuous movements, rotational and flexion-extension, or as a result of a trauma. Spondylolisthesis due to these stresses on the spine could become symptomatic.

It is always to be considered that a low back pain can be caused by musculoskeletal pathologies of other districts (such as the hip, knee, ankle, or foot) that affect the biomechanic of the walk and then movements of the spine. Other important conditions may mimic a low back pain, such as abdominal aortic aneurysm.

In these conditions the surrounding structures, and above all the paravertebral muscles, are often involved, painful, and contract.

The athlete's physical examination directs the diagnosis. It is very important to test the local pain, the sensitivity, and the motility of the lower limbs and reflexes.

The first radiological exam should be a lumbosacral X-ray or dorsal-cervical X-ray if the clinic is pathognomonic in these districts. Standard X-rays is very useful to identify active injuries that could cause the symptoms and, in case of

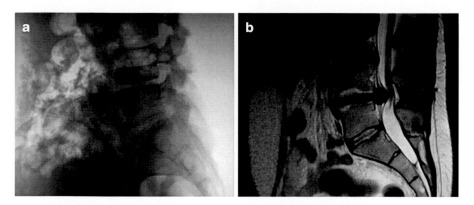

Fig. 7.1 (a) Lateral view of a low back X-ray. (b) Low back MRI shows L4–L5 disc herniation

future acute episodes, to monitor the progression of the anatomical situation with a new X-ray.

Standard X-rays might not identify a cause of low back pain.

Second-level radiological exams might be needed to complete the diagnostic: dynamics X-rays for suspected spondylolysis/spondylolisthesis or MRI (magnetic resonance imaging) in suspected stress fractures or herniated discs (Fig. 7.1).

In high-level athletes, in addition to the standard MRI, an additional MRI may be needed to make a precise diagnosis (further analyzed the clinical condition), such as the standing MRI or in other specific positions, such as seated.Vertebral fractures often have to be investigated with a computerized tomography (CT) to better evaluate the surgical indication. If conservative treatment is undertaken, usually with special spine orthosis, during the healing period, any sports activity waiting for the biological healing time can't be done.

After diagnosis if a conservative treatment is indicated, the patient starts with a variable rest period, going to identify and eliminate possible causes of back pain. Awkward postures maintained for long periods, both during sports activities and during the daily life, can lead to muscle imbalances and then to back pain. The sports gesture must be analyzed and corrected if not properly executed because it can be the cause of symptoms. Pain and inflammation could be directly treated with physical therapy (Tecar therapy, laser, ultrasounds, etc.) and drugs (NSAIDs, for short period). After the acute phase, the targets become the recovery of the movement, outside of the pain, and then strength and elasticity. Mobilization and manipulation can be useful by acting on the lumbar soft tissue. They must have the right medical indication and must be performed by a professional therapist because they can worsen the symptoms if not done correctly. The constant maintenance of muscle tone, once reinforced, is very important for the future of the back. Core stability has been reported to be essential in the prevention of back pain [2, 3].

Our national teams have within the staff, in addition to a doctor, a professional therapist to give maximum support to the athletes.

7.2   Tendon

The main function of the tendons is to transmit the muscular force to the structures to which they are connected, usually the bone segments.

The main mechanical properties of the tendons are a great mechanical strength with poor elasticity. The tendons can be stretched: up to 4% is a physiological elongation; from 4 to 8%, it comes to a partial breakage; and over 8% a complete rupture occurs.

There are several risk factors for tendon injuries that are distinct in intrinsic and extrinsic. Among the many intrinsic factors, we mention leg length discrepancy, muscular imbalances, joint's laxity, sex, and associated diseases (e.g., diabetes, autoimmune diseases). Among the extrinsic factors, we must not forget the previous injuries and local corticosteroid injections.

Tendons are often subject to overuse injuries. Their onset is characterized by pain during or after sport activity, exacerbated by palpation on it. Swelling could be present. Pain could disappear after the warm-up or can be borne by the athletes in the early stage of the injury. Continuous stresses, and overuse, lead to interfere with the healing process and leave the injury to progress.

Tendon pathology is divided into three stages. The first is the reactive tendinopathy characterized by a noninflammatory response of the tendon cells which increase the thickening of the tendon. It could be caused by a direct trauma or acute stress in young people. If the disease continues over time, the first structural alterations (second stage, tendon dysrepair) up to the degenerative tendinopathy (third stage), in which the matrix and cells continue the degenerative process and increased the fibrous tissue in the tendon and also the risk of rupture, begin to occur. Tendons that have had a lot of active episodes of tendinopathy occur more thickened, compared to the contralateral. The paratenonitis is the inflammation of the paratenon usually due to a friction over a bony prominence. Tendonitis is an uncommon inflammation of the tendon.

Rest and ice are the first treatment. It could be associated with physical therapy (laser, ultrasounds, etc.). When the acute phase is finished, the treatment continues with the recovery of the movement and the introduction of eccentric and stretching exercises.

At the muscle-tendon level, a specific work is essential. Athletes can work with iso-inertial machines: skiers report similar feelings to those found on the snow.

Initial conservative treatment has also the purpose of avoiding the surgical intervention, subcutaneous rupture of the tendon, and recurrences (by setting an appropriate preventive program that must be maintained in the future).

Surgical treatment should be done in the end stage of the tendon's pathology (third stage) to stimulate bleeding and healing with scarifications.

In young athletes the insertional tendinopathy must be differentiated from osteochondritis (e.g., Osgood-Schlatter disease) [2, 3].

The chronic tendinopathies that we found in past seasons (data from FISI, Italian Winter Sports Federation) usually affect the peroneal tendons, the tibialis anterior tendon, the Achilles tendon, the quadriceps tendon, and the rotator cuff tendons.

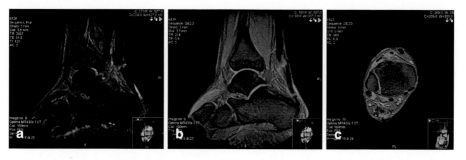

Fig. 7.2 Magnetic resonance imaging (MRI) of an ankle with an Achilles tendon rupture. (**a, b**) Sagittal view. (**c**) Axial view

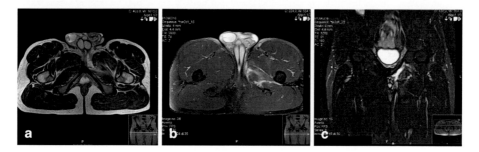

Fig. 7.3 Magnetic resonance imaging (MRI) of a pelvis with a disinsertion from the superior pubic ramus of the pectineus muscle and of the adductor longus. (**a, b**) Axial view. (**c**) Coronal view

Chronic tendinopathies can lead to tendon rupture, and the trauma's energy required for a complete lesion is frequently reduced in energy compared to acute lesions on healthy tendons. As in acute lesions, a complete tendon rupture has surgical indications in almost all cases (Fig.7.2).

Over the last 10 years, we have had complete tendon lesions that mainly affected the Achilles tendon and the adductors (data from FISI, Italian Winter Sports Federation). The surgical tenorrhaphy, or reinsertion, of the tendon has allowed the athletes to return to the elite sport activity in just a few months, without sequelae (Fig. 7.3).

7.3 Other Overuse Injuries

Skiing is a sport that overloaded the joints. A study done in healthy athletes with Tc-99m MDP bone scintigraphy has shown that joints were more stressed during the ski season. Bone scintigraphy could evaluate the joint damage even if a symptomatology is not present [4].

There were boot-related soft tissue injuries. Malleolar and adventitial bursitis could develop by chronic frictions and traumas on the lower leg due to the boot. X-rays show the swelling of the soft tissue, and MRI, or ultrasound (US), shows the content of the bursae [5]. One reason may be the use of too rigid or new boots.

Chronic injuries to the subcutaneous tissue could cause inflammatory reactions that end in the formation of a lesion that was composed by fibrosis and fat necrosis. The common localization of this pseudotumor is the lateral surface of the tibia due to the friction between the peroneal tendons-muscles, the fibula, and the boot [5].

It was reported a ski boot compression syndrome due to an anterior compression of the boot tongue at the ankle causing neuritis of the deep peroneal nerve and tenosynovitis of the extensor tendon. The treatment of this pathology is conservative and requires a reduction of the boot's compression at the ankle [6].

Pain or other symptoms persistent over time, especially if they are present even at night, should not be underestimated and require a thorough diagnostic study to rule out the presence of benign or malignant tumors.

References

1. Spörri J, Kröll J, Fasel B, Aminian K, Müller E (2016) Course setting as a prevention measure for overuse injuries of the back in alpine ski racing: a kinematic and kinetic study of giant slalom and slalom. Orthop J Sports Med 4(2):2325967116630719
2. Brukner P (2012) Brukner and Khan's clinical sports medicine. McGraw-Hill, North Ryde
3. Canale ST, Beaty JH (2012) Campbell's operative orthopaedics, XI edn. Elsevier Health Sciences, Philadelphia
4. Varoğlui E, Yildirim M, Gürsoy R, Seven B, Uslus H, Çoğalgil Ş, Kiyici F (2014) Tc-99m MDP bone scintigraphy in the evaluation of the joint damage in asymptomatic alpine ski racers. Turk J Med Sci 44(2):343–346
5. Deady LH, Salonen D (2010 Nov) Skiing and snowboarding injuries: a review with a focus on mechanism of injury. Radiol Clin N Am 48(6):1113–1124
6. Lindenbaum BL (1979) Ski boot compression syndrome. Clin Orthop Relat Res 140:109–110

Chapter 8
Prevention of Overuse Injuries in Alpine Skiers

Roberto Manzoni, Enea Bortoluz, and Alberto Sugliano

Abstract The prevention of overuse injuries is fundamental for sports physicians working with elite athletes. The knowledge of the most frequent types of injuries and the leading mechanisms are key steps to reach this goal. The correct collection and management of the data has also to be considered.

8.1 Introduction

Alpine skiing is defined as "the fastest non-motorised sport on Earth" as well as "the riskiest sport undertaken by man". Unfortunately, the fun of skiing is closely associated with a high risk of injury.

Considering the settings where alpine skiing has its highest expression—the World Cup, World Championships and Olympic Games—it can be seen that injury rates have always fluctuated, with peaks due to changes in equipment or slope grooming and periods of low incidence rates due to athletes adapting to the changes and adopting safer strategies to tackle the slope.

This peculiarity definitely shifts the focus of attention from external, performance-related factors to internal factors pertaining to the athlete and to his or her training, development and "anthropological" adaptation.

8.1.1 State of Play

In consideration of the numerous injuries sustained by its members, during the 2006–2007 season, the FIS, in collaboration with the department of research of the University of Oslo and the University of Salzburg, set up the FIS ISS (FIS Injuries

R. Manzoni (✉) • E. Bortoluz • A. Sugliano
National Alpine Ski Team, Italian Winter Sport Federation, Milan, Italy
e-mail: roberto.manzoni2014@gmail.com

© Springer International Publishing AG 2018
H. Schoenhuber et al. (eds.), *Alpine Skiing Injuries*, Sports and Traumatology,
https://doi.org/10.1007/978-3-319-61355-0_8

Surveillance System) with the aim of better understanding the mechanisms of injury and devising preventive measures to protect the athletes' health.

A 2009 paper by Florenes et al. provided a detailed retrospective analysis of the 2006–2007 and 2007–2008 World Cup seasons. The paper reports that almost 80% of professional skiers have, during the course of their career, sustained at least one severe injury, defined as an injury resulting in absence from training and competition for at least 28 days. Another major finding is the 36% overall injury rate, much higher compared to previous seasons, and the 38% rate of severe injuries, definitely higher than in other sports.

The 2014 publication by Bere, "A systematic video analysis of 69 injury cases in World Cup alpine skiing", identifies five categories of factors that expose athletes to a greater risk of injury: equipment, snow and weather conditions, speed, the piste and the competitors' athletic performance.

An analysis of these elements clearly shows that everything that characterises alpine skiing races is a potential source of danger, such that the regulations were modified to account for these factors and attempt to limit the risk. However, although recent years have seen many changes to the regulations regarding piste safety, piste marking and equipment, injuries unfortunately continue to be common in this sport.

8.1.2 Focus on Injury

To better understand the mechanisms of injury, video analyses have been successfully used to characterise knee injuries, i.e. the most common injuries in skiers accounting for over half of all injuries. However, as regards overuse problems, we are still very far from having clear data.

Studies carried out in 2015 demonstrate that there is a major difference between the number of injuries occurring in technical and speed disciplines, with special slalom recording 18% fewer injuries than the other disciplines. Giant slalom, despite being classified by FIS as a technical discipline, has very similar injury rates to the high-speed disciplines, with a difference of only 2% between downhill, super giant and giant slalom.

This could be explained by the fact that giant slalom has the highest recorded ground reaction forces, according to Gilgien's study, combined with the logical deduction that the ground reaction forces will increase with a smaller turning radius—and high speed—placing the athlete in extreme situations in terms of imbalance management, which can easily result in a loss of balance and a subsequent fall.

Moreover, it has been reported that the majority of accidents occur in the last quarter of the competition, when neuromuscular fatigue is high exposing the system to higher risk.

8.1.3 FIS Intervention

One intervention put in place by FIS in an attempt to limit accidents involved the athletes' equipment and in particular a change in the skis' turn radius. In theory, this change was meant to reduce the possibility of completing a carved turn without skidding, by imposing a lateral skid and a decrease in speed. However, Sporri's 2015 study shows that the values of anterior flexion of the trunk, lateral flexion, rotation on the body's longitudinal axis and ground reaction forces were virtually unaffected by the new equipment and, according to the athletes, the fatigue necessary for good performance levels had increased.

Sporri's study also presents other important data regarding skiing-related overuse and degenerative problems, such as low back pain.

8.1.4 Low Back Pain

The incidence of acute and/or chronic low back pain, based on interviews of the top 40 World Cup athletes, is very high, reaching 31% among males and no less than 41% among females. This incidence is more than double the values recorded for the healthy population of the same age.

In addition, according to the international guidelines on low back pain, anterior flexion, lateral flexion and rotation associated with a load—in skiing represented by gravity and ground reaction forces—tend to overload the vertebral discs exposing skiers to musculoskeletal injury.

To better understand low back pain in skiers, it is interesting to read a document issued by the Canadian Paediatric Society in 2009 which states that low back pain in youths needs to be managed differently from that of adults since their musculoskeletal system is still developing. The major risk factors include (1) muscular imbalances due to rapid bone growth and limited soft tissue flexibility; (2) structural differences like the presence of cartilaginous ossification centres which, if subjected to excessive strain during frontal and lateral flexion and torsion, can alter spine morphology predisposing the individual to spondylolysis; and (3) last but not least, inappropriate training loads and quality. The authors' recommendations for injury prevention focus on properly balancing the training load in relation to the growth period by decreasing training loads and concentrating on correct technique to promote motor control.

On the topic of motor control, it is worth mentioning the studies by Panjabi, Hides and Richardson which, although dating back to the early 1990s, remain the cornerstones of research in this field and as such are constantly cited in the recent literature.

In 1996, Hides reported that after the first episode of low back pain, the multifidus is unable to recover its full function independently despite spontaneous symptom remission and that at 10 weeks there is a clear decline in multifidus muscle tone. This, together with Gardner-Morse's findings, highlights how a 10% decline in tone can affect the muscle's stabilising function. These data prepared the way for a possible explanation of the low back pain relapse.

O'Sullivan in 1997 further developed the work done by Panjabi in 1992. Panjabi had explained that spinal instability can be identified as an area of laxity around the neutral zone which is more extensive than the symptoms ascribable to the single passive stabilisers and less extensive than those ascribable to dysfunction of the overall force of the more superficial mobiliser muscles. Instability is therefore considered an inability of the stabilising systems of the spine to maintain the neutral zone within its physiological limits.

O'Sullivan expands on these concepts and notes that the co-contractions of the deep abdominal muscles (transversus abdominis and obliquus abdominis internus) and the multifidus, by acting on the thoracolumbar fascia, are the main stabilisers of the neutral zone. Abnormality of the passive structures, such as spondylolysis and/or spondylolisthesis, requires an increase of the neuromotor system to control motor dynamics. He concludes by stating that in a setting of spinal instability, the control group, which did not undergo any programme of stabilising exercises and instruction to incorporate the skills acquired in daily life, had markedly negative outcomes.

In 2005 Hicks defined low back pain as a deviation of the lumbar-pelvic complex from its native physiological and anatomical state. In parallel, consistent with Richardson, he mentions "core training" as a method to facilitate the co-contraction of the deep abdominal muscles (transversus abdominis and obliquus abdominis internus) and multifidus which needs to be integrated into exercises and functional activities.

Stabilising exercises or "core training" are considered the treatment of choice for segmental vertebral instability, which is identified by a series of tests well described by Corkery et al.'s 2014 paper entitled "An exploratory examination of the association between altered lumbar motor control, joint mobility and low back pain in athletes".

The most significant tests to select those patients most likely to benefit from a conservative approach are:

• Assessment of lumbar ROM
• Assessment of hip ROM especially in internal rotation
• Passive SLR (straight leg raise)
• Active SLR with one leg or two legs simultaneously
• Identification of aberrant movements during ROM, such as "painful arc", "Gower's sign" and inversion of lumbar-pelvic rhythm
• Trendelenburg test
• Beighton ligamentous laxity scale

Among these tests, the SLR plus two-leg SLR associated with the Trendelenburg test are the most sensitive for assessing motor control.

In addition to this sensitive test battery for selecting those subjects with low back pain likely to respond better to motor control exercises, it should be noted that there is a close correlation between results on the Functional Movement Screen (FMS) tests and previous episodes of low back pain that may have altered the individual's general movement pattern.

Based on this view, it is clear that the athlete with low back pain requires a comprehensive assessment in order to institute the most suitable treatment allowing a reasonably fast return to play.

In conclusion, an interesting systematic review by Scheepers in 2015 analysed studies published between 1970 and 2013 in an attempt to answer the question "what intervention is to be preferred to guarantee a fast return to sports?". The study concluded that, for adult athletes for whom conservative treatment has proved ineffective, stabilisation surgery may be considered to enable return to sports, although to date there are no clear data on the quality of post-surgery sporting performances.

8.1.5 Prevention: The Concept

The issue of prevention has been widely addressed. A variety of classifications have been used to organise this complex topic; qualifiers such as "active" and "passive", "direct" and "indirect" and "primary", "secondary" and "tertiary" are combined with the term "prevention" to define the actions that can be undertaken to analyse, understand and contrast both chronic and acute sports injuries.

Recent studies conclude that prevention is an extremely complex phenomenon. Much effort is still required to gain an in-depth understanding of the processes resulting in injury, an understanding that goes beyond the mere biomechanics of the event—just as the adoption of any practice isolated from the overall context (warming up, stretching, proprioceptive exercises, etc.) does not appear to be decisive. To approach prevention coherently, information on the mechanism of injury needs to be incorporated within a model where the study of internal and external risk factors is central to modifying risk.

A recent review by Bahr and Krosshaug, "Understanding injury mechanisms: a key component of preventing injuries in sport", confirms that anterior cruciate ligament lesions are a growing cause of concern during both the chronic and the acute phase. They state that the use of specific training programmes may reduce the incidence of such injuries, but that we still do not know the programme components that are key to prevention or how the exercises work to reduce the risk. The commonly used programmes are limited by an inadequate understanding of the causes of injury. The authors therefore recommend a research model developed around four points (Fig. 8.1).

The global model should account for risk factors related to the sport and the environment (external) and those related to the athlete (internal) (Figs. 8.2 and 8.3).

Another major publication, "Research approaches to describe the mechanisms of injuries in sport: limitations and possibilities", by Krosshaug et al. proposes a multifactorial analysis of injuries according to the following model (Fig. 8.4).

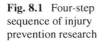

Fig. 8.1 Four-step sequence of injury prevention research

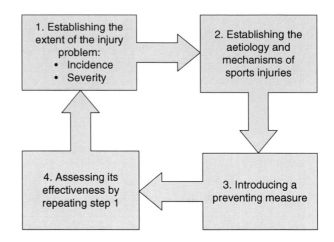

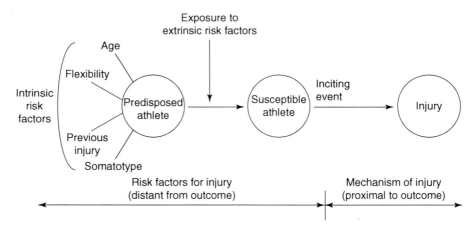

Fig. 8.2 Complex interaction between internal and external risk factors leading to an inciting event and resulting in injury

The advantage of this model is to accommodate the strengths and weaknesses of each sector of research and highlight the contribution of each to understanding and preventing sporting accidents.

The position of the federation and working group is in favour of this type of approach. The project presented for long-term athlete development (LTAD) is aimed at developing adequate motor skills for the practice of this complex discipline. Evidence-based teamwork, starting from the motor tests, enables us to customise athlete training loads and monitor the athlete's health through the use of instruments and scales to measure and assess fatigue. Instruments for training monitoring support rational working methods.

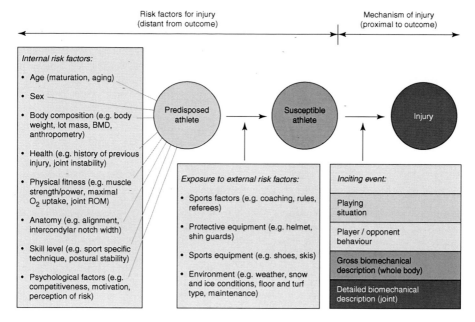

Fig. 8.3 Comprehensive model for injury causation. *BMD* body mass density, *ROM* range of motion

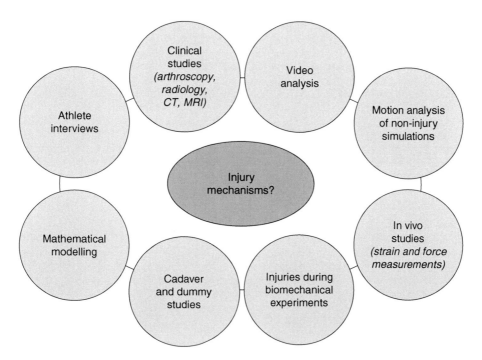

Fig. 8.4 Research approaches to describe the mechanisms of injuries in sports

Further Reading

Bere T, Flørenes TW, Krosshaug T, Haugen P, Svandal I, Nordsletten L, Bahr R (2014) A systematic video analysis of 69 injury cases in World Cup alpine skiing. Scand J Med Sci Sports 24(4):667–677

Meeuwisse WH, Tyreman H, Hagel B, Emery C (2007) A dynamic model of etiology in sport injury: the recursive nature of risk and causation. Clin J Sport Med 17(3):215–219

Bahr R, Krosshaug T (2005) Understanding injury mechanisms: a key component of preventing injuries in sport. Br J Sports Med 39(6):324–329

Krosshaug T, Andersen T, Olsen O, Myklebust G, Bahr R (2005) Research approaches to describe the mechanisms of injuries in sport: limitations and possibilities. Br J Sports Med 39(6):330–339

Hébert-Losier K, Holmberg HC (2013) What are the exercise-based injury prevention recommendations for recreational alpine skiing and snowboarding? A systematic review. Sports Med 43(5):355–366

Hegedus EJ, McDonough S, Bleakley C, Cook CE, Baxter GD (2015) Clinician-friendly lower extremity physical performance measures in athletes: a systematic review of measurement properties and correlation with injury, part 1. The tests for knee function including the hop tests. Br J Sports Med 49(10):642–648

Hegedus EJ, McDonough S, Bleakley C, Cook CE, Baxter GD (2015) Clinician-friendly lower extremity physical performance tests in athletes: a systematic review of measurement properties and correlation with injury. Part 2—the tests for the hip, thigh, foot and ankle including the star excursion balance test. Br J Sports Med 49(10):649–656

Tarara DT, Fogaca LK, Taylor JB, Hegedus EJ (2016) Clinician-friendly physical performance tests in athletes part 3: a systematic review of measurement properties and correlations to injury for tests in the upper extremity. Br J Sports Med 50(9):545–551

Spörri J, Kröll J, Fasel B, Aminian K, Müller E (2016) Course setting as a prevention measure for overuse injuries of the back in alpine ski racing. A kinematic and kinetic study of giant slalom and slalom. Orthop J Sports Med 4(2):2325967116630719

Schmitt K-U, Hörterer N, Vogt M, Frey WO, Lorenzetti S (2016) Investigating physical fitness and race performance as determinants for the ACL injury risk in alpine ski racing. BMC Sports Sci Med Rehabil 8:23

Shultz SJ, Schmitz RJ, Benjaminse A, Chaudhari AM, Collins M, Padua DA (2012) ACL research retreat VI: an update on ACL injury risk and prevention. J Athl Train 47(5):591–603

Flørenes TW, Bere T, Nordsletten L, Heir S, Bahr R (2009) Injuries among male and female World Cup alpine skiers. Br J Sports Med 43(13):973–978

Corkery MB, O'Rourke B, Viola S, Yen SC, Rigby J, Singer K, Thomas A (2014) An exploratory examination of the association between altered lumbar motor control, joint mobility and low back pain in athletes. Asian J Sports Med 5(4):e24283

Chapter 9
Musculoskeletal Disorders Among Elite Alpine Skiing Racers

Gianluca Melegati

Abstract During races, forces and accelerations must be contrasted with the use of skiing's techniques and muscles strength to ski faster and safely. Therefore, muscular injuries can negatively affect performances.

Although not a frequent occurrence during alpine skiing competitions, muscular injuries are nonetheless possible because of the very nature of the sport, where the forces are high and total loads can exceed gravity acceleration by several times, resulting in massive stress being placed on the athlete's muscular-tendinous structures.

During World Cup races, acceleration values of almost 4G are reached during curves, which translate into forces greater than 300 kg being developed on the outside leg of an 80-kg skier during a high-speed curve.

Besides adopting a correct technique and keeping the outside leg distended, to withstand such forces, the athlete must have adequate strength, which needs to be built up in the gym during summer training and maintained during the winter season.

In elite skiing, physical training plays a central role in improving sport performance and preventing injuries. Training in the gym places considerable stress on the bones, muscles and joints with a risk of acute or overload injuries at the muscular or muscular-tendinous levels.

In addition to the muscle injuries occurring during indoor or outdoor training sessions, other, more severe muscle injuries can result from falls while training or competing on the slopes.

Modern skis, with their deep sidecuts, develop a very aggressive ski-snow interaction, making it very difficult for the athlete to change trajectory once the ski has started to carve. This situation contributes significantly to increasing the risk of injury in high-speed disciplines [1].

G. Melegati
Department of Rehabilitation I, Galeazzi Orthopaedic Institute—IRCCS, Milan, Italy
e-mail: gianluca@melegati.it

© Springer International Publishing AG 2018   91
H. Schoenhuber et al. (eds.), *Alpine Skiing Injuries*, Sports and Traumatology,
https://doi.org/10.1007/978-3-319-61355-0_9

Falls often result in straining muscle groups that have been stressed to the limit of their load tolerance, especially in situations where the legs are spread apart, because of the long, unfavourable lever arm represented by the ski itself. In some cases, there may be extensive tears of the muscle structures around the pelvic girdle, at times with very serious consequences.

The physical characteristics of muscle enable it to absorb energy, and a lesion occurs when the energy developed exceeds this intrinsic capacity. Although there are numerous classifications of muscle injury, the most commonly used is the one proposed by Reid in 1992, which divides injuries into indirect trauma and direct trauma injuries [2].

Indirect trauma injuries:

- Exercise-induced muscle soreness
- Muscle lesions:

  - GRADE I: local damage to the fibrils and filaments with no loss of continuity of the affected muscle
  - GRADE II: interruption of a number of muscle fibres without involvement of a grossly recognisable portion of the muscle belly
  - GRADE III: rupture of a large portion of the muscle belly with clinically evident loss of continuity in muscle structure

  Direct trauma injuries or contusions:

  - Intermuscular haematoma
  - Intramuscular haematoma

- Avulsions:

  - Bony
  - Apophyseal
  - Muscular

The structures that are particularly exposed to the risk of indirect injury include muscle-tendon junctions, because of their limited extensibility and the abrupt reduction in local circulation in the tendon compared with the muscle, and biarticular muscles, especially those containing a greater proportion of type 2, fast-twitch fibres, such as the knee flexors or the hamstrings [3–5].

The severity of the clinical and functional picture in indirect injuries is correlated with the extent of tissue damage (Table 9.1).

Table 9.1 Clinical and functional picture of muscle injuries due to indirect trauma

Grade	Pain and contracture	Swelling and effusion	Loss of range of motion	Loss of function	Recovery time (days)
Grade I	+	Minimal	Minimal	Minimal	7–20
Grade II	++	Moderate	Significant	Significant	21–50
Grade III	+++	Extensive	Complete	Complete	60–180

The above classification, despite having been widely used internationally for several decades, does not appear to be sufficiently detailed or able to identify the more specific aspects of muscle injury or to provide valuable assistance in the diagnosis of muscle injuries.

There is a clear need for a shared international terminology able to help the clinician in the diagnosis and management of muscle injuries.

The ISMULT (Italian Society of Muscle, Ligaments and Tendons) has recently proposed a modern and complete classification, which divides muscle injuries into two broad categories depending on the mechanism of onset: direct trauma and indirect trauma [6].

9.1 Direct Trauma Injuries

Caused by a contusion (impact against an opponent or a sport-related tool or a rigid structure or the ground in the case of alpine skiing) or a laceration or wound (resulting from impact against a sharp-edged structure, such as ski edges or an opponent's shoe studs, etc.).

Laceration is not further classified into subgroups; the treatment is surgical suture, and recovery times will depend on the extent and depth of the wound.

Contusion is classed as mild, moderate or severe depending on the degree of loss of function, assessed as the ability to actively perform a movement at the level of the corresponding joint.

It is important to remember that the injury should be reassessed clinically after 24 h because the pain immediately after a contusion is often disabling, and there is a risk of considering all contusions severe. On the other hand, some direct traumas may have dramatic consequences, as is the case of compartment syndromes, which require immediate surgical intervention to prevent tissue ischaemia and muscle necrosis.

9.2 Indirect Trauma Injuries

Some injuries occur without contact or collision with the ground or barriers. These are divided into nonstructural injuries, where there is no anatomically evident damage to the muscle fibres, and structural injuries, in which the fibres are damaged.

9.2.1 Nonstructural Injuries

These are the most common and also the most difficult to diagnose and treat. They account for over 50% of days of the absence from sport activity due to muscle injuries. They should not be overlooked since, if neglected, they have a tendency to evolve into structural injuries. They are divided into four subgroups:

Type 1A: caused by fatigue and, indirectly, by continuous changes in training protocols or sport surfaces or by excessive training loads.

Type 1B: caused by too many training exercises and eccentric contractions.

Type 2A: caused by often misdiagnosed spinal disorders, such as minor intervertebral defects (MID) which irritate the spinal nerve leading to altered control of muscle tone. In these cases, resolution of the muscle injury will also require treatment of the spinal disorder.

Type 2B: due to altered neuromuscular control, especially of the reciprocal inhibition mechanism by the muscle spindles. An imbalance of this mechanism can considerably affect normal muscle tone and lead to muscle disorders. This occurs when the inhibition system of the antagonist muscle is altered (e.g. diminished), and the agonist muscle is excessively contracted for compensation.

9.2.2 Structural Injuries

These are divided into three subgroups according to the extent of the muscular tear:

Type 3A: characterised by a minor partial tear involving one or more primary fascicles within a secondary bundle

Type 3B: characterised by a partial moderate tear involving at least one secondary bundle and with less than 50% tear surface relative to the muscle section at that location

Type 4: characterised by a subtotal tear with more than 50% tear surface relative to the muscle section at that location or a complete tear involving the entire muscle belly or the tendon-bone junction

The classification of structural injuries also includes definition of lesion site in terms of proximal (P), middle (M) or distal (D). The prognosis of proximal lesions of the hamstring muscles and rectus femoris is worse than that of injuries of the same size involving other areas of the muscle. In contrast, among lesions of the triceps surae, those affecting the distal portion carry a worse prognosis.

9.3 Trauma Mechanisms

In elite skiers, the most frequently injured muscle groups are the hamstrings and the adductors, as a result of two indirect trauma mechanisms that occur in a different manner.

In fact, when analysing indirect muscle injuries in elite alpine skiing, a distinction must be made between injuries occurring in a "pure" indirect manner—that is, without contact or collision with the ground or barriers (such as injuries occurring while running during pre-season training)—and those occurring in an indirect manner but favoured by falls which, by virtue of their dynamics, cause the muscle belly to stretch while it is contracted in an attempt to resist the injuring force. When the injuring force that lengthens the muscle belly exceeds the muscle's intrinsic capacity to develop eccentric force to resist tearing of the fibres, then an injury will occur. The severity of the injury will depend on several extrinsic factors, such as the speed, the slope, the snow conditions, the ski sidecut, the calibration of the bindings and the intrinsic factors like the athlete's fatigue, muscle strength, muscle flexibility, hydration level and falling skills.

These lesions, some of which very serious, can also extend to the pelvic girdle muscles based on the same biomechanical principles underpinning adductor injury. It is not uncommon that in falls involving a split, i.e. forced spreading apart of the legs on the frontal plane, the forces at play exceed the resistance capacity of the fibres of the muscles not only of the medial compartment but also of the chest wall, including the abdominal and oblique muscles and the internal and external rotators of the hip. Even a tear of the pelvic floor can be caused by this type of traumatic event, with serious consequences also for the organs of the abdominal cavity.

Falls in elite alpine skiing can also result in direct muscle injuries, usually involving violent contact with the frozen piste or collision with poles or protective barriers. Generally, direct traumas involve the gluteal muscles, with extensive bruising and, not infrequently, intra- or intermuscular blood collections.

Another relatively common occurrence we need to be prepared for during alpine skiing races is muscle laceration due to a cut by the ski edge, which is often highly sharpened to ensure a good hold during the race. The ski edge can act like a knife and cause deep wounds that will require prompt treatment. The cases of Bode Miller and Aksel Lund Svindal in 2015 and 2007, respectively, testify to the fact that a cutting wound is a possibility to bear in mind.

Muscle injuries occurring in a "pure" indirect manner tend to happen during preseason indoor or outdoor training sessions, in situations where running is the main component. In this case, the muscles most commonly involved are those of the posterior compartment of the thigh, i.e. the hamstrings.

Hamstring injuries have been shown to have a tendency to recur [7, 8]. In a recent epidemiological study carried out on elite footballers, Hagglund et al. reported a recurrence rate of 30% for hamstring injuries and that the most commonly involved muscle was the biceps femoris [9]. In another clinical study, Ekstrand et al. found that 84% of 180 hamstring injuries detected by magnetic resonance imaging involved the biceps femoris, 11% the semimembranosus and 5% the semitendinosus [10]. The biarticular nature of the biceps femoris and other muscles of the posterior compartment of the thigh makes the hamstrings prone to injury. This is supported by the fact that also other biarticular muscles such as the gastrocnemius, adductors and rectus femoris are often a site of injury during sports [11].

Complete tear of the muscle is fortunately uncommon, accounting for 1% of all hamstring injuries. Grade III injuries may affect the muscle belly or more commonly the proximal myotendinous junction and can result in an ischial avulsion fracture or detachment of the conjoined tendon at a preinsertion site. These serious injuries may be underestimated. When this occurs and a complete tear is treated inappropriately, there is a risk chronic pain and severe loss of muscle function.

Hamstring injuries are frequent in sports featuring maximum speed running, accelerations, decelerations and changes in direction [10–16]. There is evidence that 68% of hamstring injuries in professional rugby in the United Kingdom occurred during running [17].

The hamstrings extend the hip and flex the knee. In terms of strength, speed and power, the functional requirements for normal walking and jogging are less demanding than for sprinting [18]. Experimental musculoskeletal models demonstrate that the peak hamstring torque and tension occur during the late swing phase in running and that the torque increases with running speed [19]. During running or kicking, there is a marked eccentric activation of the hamstrings. Eccentric activation during the late swing phase can cause an injury since the hamstrings generate maximum tension as they lengthen to decelerate knee extension. Data on hamstring peak torque, power, electromyographic activation and length, recorded during sprinting, showed an eccentric contraction both during the late swing phase before initial contact with the ball (foot strike) and the late stance phase before the foot is raised and takeoff. Hamstring injuries are more likely to occur during the late swing phase than during the late stance phase, because during the late swing phase, they are stretched to the limit of their structural resistance [16]. Briefly, the hamstrings act eccentrically to slow knee extension during deceleration.

Moreover, deceleration during high-speed running is often associated with forward flexion of the trunk which places an eccentric overload on the hamstrings, thereby increasing tension and the risk of muscle injury.

9.4   Principles of Functional Recovery

9.4.1   Indirect Muscle Injuries

In mild strains, the muscle repairs itself through the action of mononuclear satellite cells that differentiate into myoblasts. In more severe injuries, the formation of scar repair tissue predominates, and the progression of functional recovery is essential in that it guides the correct repair of the newly formed tissue.

The repair of muscle injuries takes place in three distinct phases: acute, remodelling and functional recovery (Table 9.2) [1–20].

Table 9.2 Repair phases of a grade II strain

Acute phase	
1 Injury	0–6 h
2 Inflammatory reaction	6–24 h
3 Phagocytosis	24–48 h
Remodelling	
4 Initial repair	3–6 days
5 Advanced repair	7–14 days
Functional recovery	
6 Functional recovery	15–60 days

Immediately after the injury, an elastic compressive bandage and cryotherapy should be applied (usually for 15 min every 2 h). In this early phase, there is local bleeding, retraction of the injured myofibrils and oedema due to increased capillary permeability. The main goal of this phase is to limit initial tissue damage as much as possible.

There is no consensus on the use of compression bandages. In a recent study, Thorsson found no effectiveness for reducing haematoma extent or recovery times in 19 subjects treated with early (within 15 min) compression after thigh and calf injury compared with 20 subjects treated with only cryotherapy and leg elevation, in some cases, combined with a compression bandage applied 10–30 min after the injury occurred [21].

Normally, the clinical situation does not warrant the use of analgesics. Moreover, the use of non-steroidal anti-inflammatory drugs (NSAIDs) to reduce inflammation in fatigue-related pain and muscle strains is controversial [22]. Although biochemical and histochemical studies have found indomethacin to be effective for reducing local muscle damage [23], other studies have reported that the use of NSAIDs is best avoided in acute muscle injuries [24] and that the use of corticosteroids in the acute phase appears to hinder healing [22].

Around 24–48 h after the injury, the oedema increases, with mechanical weakening of the muscle due to macrophage invasion. This phase requires very careful management, avoiding aggressive treatments which can cause further tissue damage, prolong the inflammatory phase and delay tissue repair. Transcutaneous electrical nerve stimulation (TENS) [23] can be safely and effectively applied for early pain relief given its prominent neuroreflexive action. Ambulation with weight bearing using two Canadian crutches is allowed as tolerated based on pain. Starting from day 3, ambulation with one Canadian crutch is normally allowed, and the compression bandage is removed to permit ultrasound examination or magnetic resonance imaging. Walking without assistive devices is allowed as soon as the gait pattern has normalised, and no local pain is experienced. Restoration of the normal gait pattern can also occur in water in decreasing pool depths. The benefits of water and its hydrostatic, hydrodynamic, proprioceptive [25] and thermal effects allow early active mobilisation with all the advantages this has on the following phase of recovering joint motion.

In terms of pathological anatomy, the acute phase is followed by initial remodelling (3–6 days post-injury); initially, fibroblastic activity is characterised by the deposition of collagen. Healing is promoted by capillary neovascularisation which provides centripetal supply of the oxygen and nutrients necessary for regenerative-reparative tissue metabolism [26]. The biostimulating effect in this phase can be heightened by physical therapies such as neodymium-doped yttrium aluminium garnet (Nd-YAG) or resistive and capacitive energy transfer (TECAR) therapy [27] applied according to specific protocols based on the sonographic findings. It should, however, be noted that the use of physical therapies is not supported by an adequate body of scientific evidence. Once the gait pattern has normalised and pain is absent, a cautious programme of passive stretching can be initiated to relax the muscle fibres in the perilesional area. No massage technique is used in this phase. The first type of muscle contraction to be introduced is isometric contraction in the form of submaximal exercising below the pain threshold.

During the advanced repair phase (7–14 days post-injury), concomitant with muscle fibre regeneration, muscle tone is approximately 50% that prior to the injury. This deficit is thought to be more due to the inflammatory nature of the healing process, with oedema and pain, than to a real decrease in contractility. The risk of re-injury during this phase is high because the pain has decreased and function has improved, while the site of injury is still structurally vulnerable. Once hamstring elasticity is satisfactory, concentric isotonic exercises are started followed by submaximal eccentric exercises, both of which done against manual resistance. Maintenance or restoration of tissue elasticity involves the performance of specific passive stretching exercises. As regards the timing of stretching exercises, Bandy et al. reported that daily 30-s passive stretching sessions provide optimal results and that longer sessions up to 60 s do not produce a parallel increase in flexibility [28]. Moreover, in this phase, aerobic exercise is introduced in the form of a cycle ergometer and step machine, with running postponed to the next phase of functional recovery. Proprioceptive rehabilitation is then gradually introduced in three progressive stages: joint positioning/repositioning (cortical level), single-leg and two-leg balance training with eyes open and eyes shut (subcortical level) and dynamic reflexive stabilisation exercises and sport-specific activities (spinal level).

During the functional recovery phase (15–60 days post-injury), following collagen maturation and complete recovery of voluntary muscular control, the aim of rehabilitation is to restore strength and function. As a rule, normal gait and muscular elasticity have been recovered between the third and fourth week, and prolonged maximal isometric contraction does not elicit pain. At this stage, sonography is obtained to determine the progression of fibre remodelling in the scar tissue.

Heiser et al. recommend introducing running when the peak torque at an angular velocity of 60°/s is at least 70% that of the contralateral limb [29]. This presumes that maximal isokinetic testing has been performed which, however, may predispose the athlete to re-injury. It is important to note that isokinetic dynamometry is useful for evaluating muscle strength expressed during open kinetic chain exercise in the absence of loading. As a result, it is impossible to reproduce joint kinematics in a closed kinetic chain system with loading. This means that the test is inappropriate for assessing the role of the musculature in dynamic joint stabilisation. Aagard et al. suggested interpolating the peak eccentric torque of the hamstrings from the peak concentric torque of the quadriceps (eccentric ham/concentric quad), defining the result as the "functional ratio of the knee extensors" [30]. In this case, the peak hamstring torque is directly proportional to the angular velocity of the exercise and inversely proportional to the degree of knee flexion. In a study of professional footballers, Dauty et al. reported that an eccentric ham/concentric quad ratio less than 0.6 identified players who, although returned to play, had experienced a previous hamstring injury. However, the ratio was not predictive of future injuries [31].

Eccentric isokinetic exercise at increasing speeds (starting at 60°/s), beginning at submaximal intensity, is performed no more than three times a week, taking care to avoid any overload during those days to prevent possible muscle fatigue.

Because hamstring strain typically occurs during the eccentric phase of muscle contraction, a specific rehabilitation programme with eccentric strengthening is crucial. Exercise performed at high angular velocity is the key to the success of the rehabilitation programme. On this topic, Jonhagen et al. reported that the recurrence of hamstring strains in athletes engaging in sports characterised by high angular velocities, such as sprinters, is often due to a strength deficit in the eccentric phase [32].

Electrostimulation of the affected area is not, in our opinion, warranted during rehabilitation after a muscle strain nor are there any published studies confirming its effective utility.

Unrestricted training can start when muscle strength is at least 80% that of the contralateral limb and when prolonged running does not cause muscle fatigue.

Athletes who have sustained a hamstring strain should continue with eccentric exercising for the rest of their professional career.

The strong tendency of muscle injuries, and hamstring strains in particular, to recur poses additional challenges for the physician who will have to find the right balance between the primary need to prevent recurrences and the need to ensure rapid recovery. Return to play will depend on adequate recovery of muscle strength, resistance and flexibility, as well as on neuromuscular control.

The site and extent of muscle damage, the athlete's motivation and general psychophysical state, the appropriate rehabilitation techniques and the perfect coordination of all components of the medical staff are all factors that influence the athlete's full functional recovery.

Recurrence of an injury within 2 months after return to play is a clear sign of an inadequate rehabilitation programme.

9.4.2   Direct Muscle Injuries

High-speed falls with impact against the ski course generally cause a direct muscle injury, with compression of the muscular tissue and possible haematoma formation. The blood infiltrates the underlying tissues leading to bruises, and in some cases it collects between the damaged muscle fibres and along the intermuscular spaces.

Contusions are classified into grade II characterised by bruises, grade II characterised by haematoma and grade III with skin necrosis and possible ulceration, which may be accompanied by fever and, in more severe cases, by shock [33].

Direct muscle injuries are often considered minor injuries that are likely to resolve rapidly without consequences. However, the high speeds achieved by athletes in elite alpine skiing mean that the impact against the ground, barriers or poles can result in serious clinical conditions, with major bruising and intermuscular or intramuscular blood collections requiring ultrasound-guided drainage and very aggressive compressive treatment.

In terms of pathological anatomy, the muscle tears produced by such traumas do not essentially differ from muscle injury due to other mechanisms. Functionally, the muscle contraction caused by the trauma limits joint range of motion because of reduced muscle extensibility. On the basis of this principle, Reid proposed the following classification, indirectly related to range of motion, which is the most commonly adopted and applied given its ease of use in clinical practice [2].

1. Mild muscle injury: over 50% of range of motion
2. Moderate muscle injury: less than 50% but more than 1/3 range of motion
3. Severe muscle injury: less than 1/3 range of motion

Direct trauma is often characterised by haematoma, which may be intramuscular, intermuscular or mixed intra- and intermuscular.

Intramuscular haematoma is characterised by the structural integrity of the connective tissue fascia covering the muscle belly which acts as a barrier and confines the haematoma to the muscle [34]. This situation causes increased intramuscular pressure and capillary bed compression which counteracts the bleeding, while the resulting clinical signs and symptoms remained confined to the site of injury.

The main symptoms of intramuscular haematoma are pain during the first 72 h post-injury, decreased contractile capability and increased rigidity of the muscle.

A contusion occurring on a contracted muscle is absorbed more superficially than on a relaxed muscle, in which the haematoma will form at a deeper level because the impact results in increased intramuscular pressure which is transmitted as far as the bone [35–37].

In intermuscular haematoma the muscle fascia is damaged allowing the blood to seep between the muscle bellies and between the muscle belly and the fascia. Unlike intramuscular haematoma, intermuscular haematoma causes pain which is limited to the first 24 h post-injury [38].

Finally, in mixed intra- and intermuscular haematoma, following an initial, transient phase of increased pressure due to bleeding, the pressure decreases rapidly. Swelling due to bleeding generally appears 24–48 h after the injury, but there is no rapid increase in pressure, the swelling tends to be temporary, functional recovery is fairly rapid and healing is usually complete. The clinical diagnosis of a superficial haematoma is more straightforward because of bruising appearing on the impact zone, with swelling and impaired muscle function depending on the impact force. By contrast, a deep haematoma is clinically more difficult to diagnose. First, it is important to remember that a correct diagnosis only becomes possible 48–72 h after the injury since the haematoma may have a delayed onset. Magnetic resonance imaging and ultrasound are crucial and strongly recommended in these cases. The prognosis is good when the swelling and pain decrease, and muscle function is gradually and rapidly recovered in the first 24 h post-injury. If the swelling persists beyond 48–72 h, with gradually worsening pain and persisting functional impairment in terms of muscle stiffness and limited range of motion, the prognosis is considered negative [39]. There is very little evidence of the most appropriate physical therapy for direct traumas. Generally, clinical good sense and professional experience are able to guide the management of these cases. Care should be taken to avoid treatments involving the application of heat at least during the 5–7 days after the injury. A gradual progression of recovery is always warranted, avoiding excessive stress and working within pain-free ranges and functional limitations. In general terms, the prognosis of intermuscular haematoma is always better than that of intramuscular haematoma [39]. In the first case, early initiation of a programme to restore mobility will allow a rapid return to skiing, depending on the extent of the injury. Recovery and return to skiing after a mild injury (grade I in Reid's classification) can take 5–7 days, whereas after a grade II and III injury, it will take between 2 and 12 weeks. Intramuscular haematoma requires more careful management of functional recovery and return to sport, because of the risk of myositis ossificans. One of the most serious potential complications of inadequate management can occur if treatment is started too soon or if it is too aggressive or too conservative and does not support healing by applying loads correctly and progressively. As a rule, in the case of an intramuscular haematoma, return to sport cannot be recommended before 2–5 months after the injury [40].

References

1. Kröll J, Spörri J, Gilgien M, Schwameder H, Müller E (2016) Effect of ski geometry on aggressive ski behaviour and visual aesthetics: equipment designed to reduce risk of severe traumatic knee injuries in alpine giant slalom ski racing. Br J Sports Med 50:20–25
2. Reid DC (1992) Muscle injury: classification and healing. In: Sport injury. Assessment and rehabilitation. Churchill Livingstone, New York, pp 85–101
3. Brewer BJ (1962) Athletic injuries: musculotendinous unit. Clin Orthop 23:30
4. Agre JC, Baxter TL (1981) Strength and flexibility characteristics of collegiate soccer players. Arch Phys Med Rehabil 62:539
5. Garrett WE, Califf JC, Bassett FH (1984) Histochemical correlates of hamstring injuries. Am J Sports Med 12:98–103
6. Maffulli N, Oliva F, Frizziero A et al (2013) ISMuLT guidelines for muscle injuries. Muscles Ligaments Tendons J 3(4):241–249
7. Tsaousidis N, Zatsiorski V (1996) Two types of ball-effector interaction and their relative contribution to soccer kicking. Hum Mov Sci 15:861–876
8. Hay JG (1996) The biomechanics of sports techniques. Prentice Hall, Englewood Cliffs, NJ
9. Hagglund M, Walden M, Ekstrand J (2005) Injury incidence and distribution in elite football: a prospective study of the Danish and the Swedish top divisions. Scand J Med Sci Sports 15:21–28
10. Ekstrand J, Gillquist J (1983) Soccer injuries and their mechanism: a prospective study. Med Sci Sports Exerc 15:267–270
11. Witvrouw E, Danneels L, Asselman P et al (2003) Muscle flexibility as a risk factor for developing muscle injuries in male professional soccer players. Am J Sports Med 31:41–46
12. Volpi P, Melegati G, Tornese D et al (2004) Muscle strains in soccer: a five-year survey of an Italian major league team. Knee Surg Sports Traumatol Arthrosc 12:482–485
13. Burkett LN (1970) Causative factors of hamstring strains. Med Sci Sports Exerc 2:39–42
14. Agre JC (1985) Hamstring injuries: proposed etiologic factors, prevention and treatment. Sports Med 2:21–33
15. Stafford MG, Grana WA (1984) Hamstring/quadriceps ratios in college football players: a high velocity evaluation. Am J Sports Med 12:209–211

16. Worrell TW (1994) Factors associated with hamstring injuries. An approach to treatment and preventive measures. Sports Med 17:338–345
17. Brooks JH, Fuller CW, Kemp SP, Reddin DB (2005) Epidemiology of injuries in English professional rugby union: part 1 match injuries. Br J Sports Med 39(10):757–766
18. Orchard J, Marsden J, Lord S et al (1997) Preseason hamstring weakness associated with hamstring muscle injury in Australian footballers. Am J Sports Med 25:81–85
19. Dvorak J, Junge A, Chomiak J et al (2000) Risk factor analysis for injuries in football players. Possibilities for a prevention program. Am J Sports Med 28:S58–S68
20. Fisher BD et al (1990) Ultrastructural events following acute muscle trauma. Med Sci Sports Exerc 22:185–193
21. Thorsson O, Lilja B, Nilsson P, Westlin N (1997) Immediate external compression in the management of an acute muscle injury. Scand J Med Sci Sports 7:182–190
22. Almekinders LC (1999) Anti-inflammatory treatment of muscular injuries in sport. An update of recent studies. Sports Med 28:383–388
23. Wolf SL (1978) Perspectives on central nervous system responsiveness to transcutaneous electrical nerve stimulation. Phys Ther 58(12):1443–1449
24. Speer KP, Cavanaugh JT, Warren RF, Day L, Wickiewicz TL (1993) A role for hydrotherapy in shoulder rehabilitation. Am J Sports Med 21:850–853
25. Reynolds JF, Noakes TD, Schwellnus MP, Windt A, Bowerbank P (1995) Non-steroidal anti-inflammatory drugs fail to enhance healing of acute hamstring injuries treated with physiotherapy. S Afr Med J 85:517–522
26. Benazzo F, Barnabei G, Monti G, Ferrario A, Jelmoni GP (1989) Attuali orientamenti nella patogenesi, evoluzione e trattamento degli ematomi muscolari negli atleti. Italian J Sports Traumatol 4:273–304
27. Mondardini P, Tanzi R, Verardi L, Briglia S, Maione A, Drago E (1999) Nuove metodologie nel trattamento della patologia traumatica dell'atleta: la T.E.C.A.R. terapia. Med Sport 52:201–213
28. Bandy WD, Irion JM (1994) The effect of time on static stretch on the flexibility of the hamstring muscle. Phys Ther 74:845–850
29. Heiser TM, Weber J, Sullivan G, Clare P, Jacobs RR (1984) Prophylaxis and management of hamstring muscle injuries in intercollegiate football players. Am J Sports Med 12:368–370
30. Aagaard P, Simonsen EB, Magnusson SP, Larsson B, Dyhre-Poulsen P (1998) A new concept for isokinetic hamstring: quadriceps muscle strength ratio. Am J Sports Med 26:231–237
31. Dauty M, Potiron-Josse M, Rochcongar P (2003) Consequences et prediction des lesions musculaires des ischiojambiers a partir des parametres isocinetiques concentriques et excentriques du joueur de football professional. Ann Readapt Med Phys 46:601–606
32. Jönhagen S, Németh G, Eriksson E (1994) Hamstring injuries in sprinters. The role of concentric and eccentric hamstring muscle strength and flexibility. Am J Sports Med 22:262–266
33. Hudon MA (1996) Introduction. In: Hudson MA (ed) Sports injuries: recognition and management, 2nd edn. Oxford University Press, Oxford, pp 1–16
34. Bird S, Black N, Newton P (1997) Sport injuries. Causes, diagnosis, treatment and prevention. Stanley Thornes Ltd, Cheltenhan
35. Crisco JJ, Hentel KD, Jackson WO, Goehner K, Jokl P (1996) Maximal contraction lessens impact response in a muscle contusion models. J Biomech 29:1291–1296
36. Garret WE (1996) Muscle strain injury. Am J Sports Med 24:2–8
37. Garret WE, Safran MR, Seaber AV, Glisson RR, Ribbeck BM (1987) Biomechanical comparison of stimulated and nonstimulated skeletal muscle pilled to failure. Am J Sports Med 15:448–454
38. Klein JH (1990) Muscular hematomas: diagnosis and management. J Manip Physiol Ther 13:96–100
39. Reström P (2003) Muscle injury. In: Ekstrand J, Karlsson J, Hodson A (eds) Football medicine. Martin Dunitz, London, pp 217–228
40. Bisciotti GM (2013) Il trattamento delle lesioni muscolari. Sport e Medicina

Chapter 10
Return to Elite Alpine Sports Activity After Injury

Roberto Manzoni, Enea Bortoluz, and Alberto Sugliano

Abstract Return to sport after an injury is always a tricky and complicated process. Many roads can be undertaken to reach the goal of returning to the same competitive level. Athletes must be followed in all their steps by different professional figures who must work together.

10.1 Introduction

As previously seen, the goal of sports training is to improve the result during competition Prevention takes place at different levels: first, making sure that injury does not occur; then, in the unfortunate case it does occur, using the most adequate means and instruments for treatment and rehabilitation; finally monitoring the risk of relapse. A previous injury is known to be associated with a fourfold increase in the risk of re-injury [1, 2].

The timing of return to sport is a fairly important problem for the medical and coaching team. It is a field in which the competences of the physician, physiotherapist, technician, physical trainer and psychologist come together. In some cases even the athlete's manager will play a role [3].

The keyword is recovery. Whether following surgery or conservative treatment, recovery has many manifestations. The most important are biological, anatomical, articular, functional, technical, sporting, psychological healing. The timing and manner of return to play without restrictions are established according to criteria (not always measureable) that must take all the manifestations into account. The subject of return to play, or return to sports, is of great interest to scientific research [3–5].

R. Manzoni (✉) • E. Bortoluz • A. Sugliano
National Alpine Ski Team, Italian Winter Sport Federation, Milan, Italy
e-mail: roberto.manzoni2014@gmail.com

© Springer International Publishing AG 2018   103
H. Schoenhuber et al. (eds.), *Alpine Skiing Injuries*, Sports and Traumatology,
https://doi.org/10.1007/978-3-319-61355-0_10

10.1.1   Decision-Based Model for Return to Play

A systematic review of the literature published in 2010 and entitled "Return-to-Play in Sport: A Decision-based Model", provides a model to guide decisions on the timing of return to play for the individual athlete. It develops through three steps, the athlete's health status, the risk factors, and the decision-making process. The publication is devoted to sports medicine but it aims to guide decisions for all the satellite disciplines, such as alpine skiing, discussed in this chapter [6].

Incorporating the indications of the studies reviewed, the model considers three broad areas—medical-clinical aspects, sport- and athlete-related aspects and associated risk factors, the final decision-making process. In other words, it considers all those aspects which, combined, will influence return-to-play decisions. On the right are the details and information to be analysed in rational decision making. In all fields, the decision-making process is based on the risk-benefit ratio and is recursive, that is, repeated for each change in any single factor over time (Fig. 10.1).

The authors state that to appreciate the athlete's health status it is preferable to consider the history of the condition (or injury), the symptoms, the signs on physical examination and imaging, laboratory tests and functional tests, as well as an estimate of the biological healing time of tissues. It is recognised that this is a novel and developing approach, but there is extensive evidence documenting discrepancies between imaging data and theoretical expectations.

Below is a detailed description of the information that needs to be taken into account and that contributes to the final return-to-play (RTP) decision.

10.1.2   Step 1: Evaluation of Health Status

The subject's demographic data (e.g. sex and age) influence the health status because of hormonal factors that can affect tissue regenerative abilities.

Assessment of symptoms and their history provides very important information for identifying possible risk factors. Pain, for example, is considered an essential factor in the evaluation presumably because it is indicative of incomplete healing. Other symptoms often used by clinicians, such as stiffness or sensation of joint stability, were not explicitly addressed by the studies included in the review.

Personal medical history: the literature emphasises some aspects of the history that are related to the current injury. For example, a distinction must be made between first-time injuries and recurrent injuries. Family history and medical history can predispose an athlete to other medical conditions or injuries.

Muscle strength and joint range of motion (ROM) are almost unanimously considered criteria that heavily influence final RTP decisions.

Muscle strength should be at or near pre-injury levels, and is often measured compared to the contralateral limb. The acceptable range is 70–100%, although it

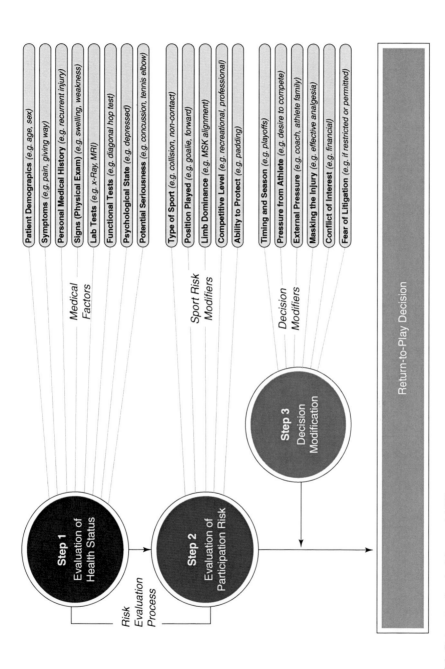

Fig. 10.1 Return-to-play decision model [6]

Table 10.1 General recommendations for each of the physical signs used by clinicians to evaluate whether an athlete should be allowed to return to play

Sign	General recommendation
Strength	At or near pre-injury levels or symmetrical with unaffected side
Range of motion	At or near pre-injury levels or symmetrical with unaffected side
Joint stability	No instability
Tenderness	Injury site should be nontender
Inflammation or swelling	No swelling or inflammation
Effusion	No effusion
Girth	No specific recommendation provided

should be noted that these references are more based on expert opinion than on scientific evidence (which is probably lacking).

Similar criteria have been proposed for ROM, specifying that terminal ROM should be pain-free.

The injury site should be functionally stable and nontender. The tissue should show no signs of inflammation or other physiological changes.

These recommendations are summarised in Table 10.1.

Laboratory tests with imaging techniques are considered highly useful for determining healing of the lesion.

Function tests. As stated above, there may be a discrepancy between biological and functional healing. To confirm recovery, it may sometimes be necessary to use sport-specific tests.

A good battery of tests will allow assessment of muscular strength, ROM, proprioception, resistance, and psychological status. Psychological confidence and readiness are positive; apprehension, fear and anxiety are associated with an increased risk of re-injury (as well as negatively affecting performance). Stability, control and ergonomic kinematics of pain-free movement, as compared to the contralateral limb give the green light to return to training and competition [6].

10.1.3 Step 2: Evaluation of Risk

The type of sport clearly entails different risks of sustaining an injury. Contact and collision sports like football and rugby or basketball have an intrinsic higher risk of acute injury. Other sports like swimming and long-distance running more often predispose to chronic conditions. Alpine skiing deserves special attention as it is a high-speed sport performed in an unstable and variable environment. RTP decisions must clearly take into account these factors as well as the sport and the athlete's limb dominance.

The competitive level would appear uninfluential. In actual fact, however, elite athletes reach higher speeds and produce greater forces and greater stresses compared with others at lower competitive level. Elite athletes are also more likely to push themselves beyond their limits in an attempt to win. As a result, they have a greater health risk.

Another aspect to be considered is whether, according to the rules of the sport, athletes are allowed to protect themselves using protective devices such as orthoses [6].

10.1.4 Step 3: Decision Modifiers

Timing and season will orientate and influence RTP decisions. The risk-benefit ratio needs to be carefully considered. Alpine skiing has a ranking calculation system which often affects decisions to request injury status or interrupt it to return to competition. Clearly, a distinction is made between minor, short-term disabilities and major injuries with over 3 months expected recovery time.

The medicolegal aspects of RTP fall to the clinician and at times the timing and manner of RTP do not coincide with those of the athlete, who may, for example, be influenced by family members, coach, or manager, or who may be at their first injury and thus unable to judge an acceptable level of risk.

Another factor evaluated by the authors is external pressure. This includes all those groups of people who may stand to benefit indirectly from the athlete's timely return to competition. The contribution deriving from the participation of these groups may be valuable or, when incompetent or intentionally misleading, it may be dangerous. In such a complex context this possible variable cannot be overlooked.

Masking an injury with medication is strongly discouraged if the athlete's well-being is a priority and running the risk of worsening the condition is not acceptable.

Conflict of interest can also potentially interfere with RTP decisions. The athlete's and the federation's best interests may not be perfectly aligned. It is the clinician's and staff's ethical and moral duty to be transparent and provide the athlete with accurate information.

Documentation and sharing of RTP decisions is also necessary as it will constitute evidence in the event of possible future litigation arising as a result of re-injury or perceived inappropriate restriction [6].

The *Italian Federation of Winter Sports* is aligned with this approach to dealing with, analysing, measuring, evaluating and deciding on the injured athlete's return to play. The model involves both the physicians of the Medical Committee and the Team of technicians, physiotherapists and physical trainers, clearly together with the athletes and their entourage.

10.1.5   Focus on Anterior Cruciate Ligament Injuries

In addition to being the most popular winter sport worldwide, alpine skiing is, unfortunately, also the sport that carries the highest risk of injury.

Looking specifically at the most common and disabling injury, we find that, according to studies cited by the International Federation, the knee is the most commonly involved body part, with more than 58% of all injuries. The most frequent diagnosis is rupture of the anterior cruciate ligament (ACL), accounting for 35.6% of all injuries and 67.9% of surgical operations on the knee [7, 8].

In terms return to play, can a top-level skier with rupture and subsequent surgical reconstruction of the ACL return to pre-injury levels of performance?

An important retrospective study (descriptive, epidemiological), entitled "Return to Sport among French Alpine Skiers after an Anterior Cruciate Ligament Rupture. Results From 1980 to 2013", attempted to answer this question using an original and accurate approach. The study sample consisted of French skiers who competed on the French national alpine skiing teams between 1980 and 2013 [9].

A first important consideration is that the likelihood of returning to pre-injury performance levels has been reported to depend more on the athlete's personality, emotional and cognitive status than on the quality of the functional knee reconstruction. The study was conducted with very rigorous tools and methods. The inclusion of the sample, and control group, the reference outcomes, the performance indexes were all well correlated. The results show that all the athletes resumed their career after the injury, in some cases even with improved competitive achievements. Age appears to have a role, with the likelihood of achieving improved performance being greater when the injury and subsequent recovery occur before the age of 25 years (statistically the age at peak performance both for males and females), and is better for women. Therefore, it is indeed possible to return to competitive sport and even to improve performance levels [10, 11].

What are the rehabilitation guidelines and the criteria for return to play?

10.1.6   Rehabilitation Guidelines and RTP Criteria Following ACL Reconstruction

From "Suggestions From the Field for Return-to-Sport Rehabilitation Following Anterior Cruciate Ligament Reconstruction: Alpine Skiing" [12].

A rehabilitation programme for the most successful (and safest) recovery of the athlete must be based on the best scientific evidence and have a clear sport-specific connotation.

The rehabilitation programme consists of three phases: post-surgery, sport-specific training and return-to-sport training. Below we report the goals to be achieved and the criteria used to determine progression.

The initial post-surgery phase following ACL reconstruction (general reconstruction without complications or associated lesions) occurs between 4–6 weeks after surgery. It should be aimed at biological tissue healing, joint mobility and restoration of gait.

TABLE 1	CRITERIA FOR PROGRESSION AND GOALS OF REHABILITATION FOLLOWING ANTERIOR CRUCIATE LIGAMENT RECONSTRUCTION

Minimum Criteria to Progress to Advanced Functional Rehabilitation
1. Minimal joint effusion
2. Normal, symmetrical gait
3. Symmetrical and functional quadriceps recruitment
4. No episodes of giving way or apprehension with closed-kinetic-chain activities or activities of daily living
5. Passive range of motion symmetrical/functional extension, flexion to 90% of contralateral side

Goals of Advanced Phase of Rehabilitation (Weeks 4-6)
1. Restore muscular strength in functional range of motion
2. Optimize neuromuscular control/balance/proprioception
3. Optimize core dynamic stability
4. Improve cardiovascular fitness

Minimum Criteria to Progress to Sport-Specific Training Phase
1. Symmetrical double-limb squat held at 60˚ for 30 seconds
2. Symmetrical single-limb squat to 30˚ without varus/valgus compensations

Goals of Sport-Specific Training Phase (Weeks 6-16)
1. Pass functional sports test
2. Strength within 85% or greater of contralateral side
3. Improve cardiovascular fitness

Minimum Criteria to Advance to Return-to-Sport Phase
1. Pass functional sports test
2. Thigh girth within 1 cm of contralateral side, measured at 15 cm above patella
3. Cleared by physician: satisfactory exam

Goals of Return-to-Sport Phase (Weeks 16-24)
1. Achieve maximal neuromuscular control, endurance, strength, power, and balance
2. Safely return athlete to full competitive level while protecting reconstructed anterior cruciate ligament graft

The minimum criteria for initiating the first phase of rehabilitation are:

- no joint effusion
- normal gait
- symmetrical and functional muscular recruitment
- active and passive knee extension equal to contralateral knee
- no episode of giving way or apprehension during activities of daily living
- passive range of motion to 90% of healthy knee

The recommendations are:

• strong isometric contractions of the quadriceps muscles even with the use of electrical stimulation and biofeedback
• exercises for neuromuscular and proprioceptive control
• exercises for orthostatic balance
• closed kinetic chain activities
• exercises for the contralateral leg and trunk (core)
• exercises for cardiovascular fitness (also to provide an emotional stimulus and a sense of well-being)

Minimal criteria to progress to the sport-specific training phase:

• Symmetrical double-limb squat held at 60° for 30″
• Symmetrical single-limb squat to 30° without frontal-plane compensations

The goals of sport-specific training phase (weeks 6–16):

• pass the sport-specific test battery (see Sect. 3.10 of Chap. 3)
• muscle strength, as measured with various ergometers, should not show more than 25% deficit compared to the contralateral limb
• continue to improve cardiovascular fitness

Minimum criteria to progress to return-to-sport phase:

• good scores on previously mentioned sport-specific tests
• thigh girth, as measured 15 cm above patella, should be within 1 cm of healthy side
• satisfactory clinical examination

Goals of return-to-sport phase (week 16–24):

• achieve maximal neuromuscular control, endurance, strength, power, and balance
• safe return of athlete to pre-injury competitive level

The next step is the return-to-ski programme. This involves a taxonomic progression in difficulty and speed, under the supervision of a trainer-coach. The athlete will progress from skiing on groomed terrain without obstacles to skiing on a training course with gates. The variables are the terrain, the slope, the type of snow, the piste, the discipline, the percentage of technical intensity and the workload. All this will continue until full return to alpine skiing provided that no significant symptoms arise.

The review ends with an assessment form entitled "Sport test: functional assessment, return to sport" consisting of a series of tests to evaluate the anatomical ergonomics, the asymmetries, the effectiveness and efficiency of various movements, from more static to more dynamic movements such as isometric squat and dynamic squat, forward and backward running, jumping. Lateral movements and direction changes with control of knee valgus, together with other movements, are those that most influence judgement. Strength, endurance, control and agility are the findings that lead to a judgement of fitness to return to training for competition [12].

10.2   Conclusions

Rehabilitation following ACL reconstruction has undergone profound changes over the past 25 years. Despite the major efforts and energy invested by researchers there are no objective standardised criteria to accurately assess an athlete's ability to progress through the final stages of rehabilitation and achieve a safe return to sport.

Return-to-sport decisions will therefore be guided by clinical algorithmic reasoning that will take into account the athlete's unique characteristics as well as all the measureable factors and definable criteria discussed so far.

References

1. Paterno MV, Schmitt LC, Ford KR, Rauh MJ, Myer GD, Huang B, Hewett TE (2010) Biomechanical measures during landing and postural stability predict second anterior cruciate ligament injury after anterior cruciate ligament reconstruction and return to sport. Am J Sports Med 38(10):1968–1978
2. Myklebust G, Bahr R (2005) Return to play guidelines after anterior cruciate ligament surgery. Br J Sports Med 39(3):127–131
3. Myer GD, Paterno MV, Ford KR, Quatman CE, Hewett TE (2006) Rehabilitation after anterior cruciate ligament reconstruction: criteria-based progression through the return-to-sport phase. J Orthop Sports Phys Ther 36(6):385–402
4. Myer GD, Paterno MV, Ford KR, Hewett TE (2008) Neuromuscular training techniques to target de cits before return to sport after anterior cruciate ligament reconstruction. J Strength Cond Res 22(3):987–1014
5. Nordahl B (2011) Return to elite alpine sports activity after an anterior cruciate ligament injury. Ski high school students' experiences. Master Thesis, Linnaeus University
6. Creighton DW, Shrier I, Shultz R, Meeuwisse WH, Matheson GO (2010) Return-to-play in sport: a decision-based model. Clin J Sport Med 20(5):379–385
7. Nordahl B, Sjöström R, Westin M, Werner S, Alricsson M (2014) Experiences of returning to elite alpine skiing after ACL injury and ACL reconstruction. Int J Adolesc Med Health 26(1):69–77
8. Smith FW, Rosenlund EA, Aune AK, MacLean JA, Hillis SW (2004) Subjective functional assessments and the return to competitive sport after anterior cruciate ligament reconstruction. Br J Sports Med 38(3):279–284
9. Haida A, Coulmy N, Dor F et al (2016) Return to sport among French alpine skiers after an anterior cruciate ligament rupture. Results from 1980 to 2013. Am J Sports Med 44(2):324–330
10. Ardern CL, Webster KE, Taylor NF, Feller JA (2011) Return to the preinjury level of competitive sport after anterior cruciate ligament reconstruction surgery. Two-thirds of patients have not returned by 12 months after surgery. Am J Sports Med 39(3):538–543
11. Grassi A, Zaffagnini S, Marcheggiani Muccioli GM, Neri MP, Della Villa S, Marcacci M (2015) After revision anterior cruciate ligament reconstruction, who returns to sport? A systematic review and meta-analysis. Br J Sports Med 49(20):1295–1304
12. Kokmeyer D, Wahoff M, Mymern M (2012) Suggestions from the field for return-to-sport rehabilitation following anterior cruciate ligament reconstruction: alpine skiing. J Orthop Sports Phys Ther 42(4):313–325

Chapter 11
Role of Ski Equipment on Injury Rate

Paolo Capitani, Gabriele Thiébat, Andrea Panzeri, and Herbert Schoenhuber

Abstract The history of the specifications for competition equipment and races from 1985 to our days is full of changes. These are about competition equipments (skis, bindings, ski boots, etc.) and also courses (e.g., International Ski Federation rules). In this chapter we try to match these changes with the different types of injuries of the Italian Alpine Ski Team during years.

Ski equipments help to ski faster and, at the same time, their main role is to reduce the risk of injuries. Performance in alpine ski racers is affected by lots of elements including biomechanics. In slalom (SL) and giant slalom (GS) due to the characteristics of the slopes, the skiing style is aimed at reducing the amount of dissipated speed at every turn. Therefore athletes try to early start turns and carve instead of skid. In downhill (DH) aerodynamic is the key point. Ski equipments must be inserted in this context, never forgetting safety [1, 2].

Skidding and carving had similar stress loading of the knee [3].

There were a lot of intrinsic and extrinsic factors which could lead to injuries in alpine ski. Acting only on one of these elements couldn't completely manage whole problems: a directional multidisciplinary approach is the correct solution to find the right direction in injury prevention, taking into account that not all these risk factors have the same weight in modifying the risk of injuries. The set of skis, boots, and binding represented an indivisible whole which, according to experts, transmitted the forces in all their energy making it difficult to control in case of loss of balance. Experts reported that with modern equipment less speed is lost during a curve than in the past. However maintaining a consistently high speed, the athlete's concentration paradoxically is reduced [4].

The ski binding release is the weakest link in the safety chain. The new skis and technical equipment, which transmit a lot of energy back to the athlete while skiing,

P. Capitani (✉) • G. Thiébat • A. Panzeri • H. Schoenhuber
Sport Traumatology Centre, IRCCS Istituto Ortopedico Galeazzi,
Via Riccardo Galeazzi 4, 20161 Milano, Italy
e-mail: paolocapitani.dr@gmail.com

© Springer International Publishing AG 2018
H. Schoenhuber et al. (eds.), *Alpine Skiing Injuries*, Sports and Traumatology,
https://doi.org/10.1007/978-3-319-61355-0_11

have much improved performance, but doing so they have made more difficult the control of the skis. It always needs the maximum concentration, strength, reactivity and attention by the athlete.

Taking into account all risk factors and exposure in giant slalom, super giant slalom (SG), and downhill, they were dangerous in the same way in facilitating injuries. High speed was the key to understand a lot of the factors involved. Higher speed means the more time in jump, the more force of impact in case of fall and fewer preparation time for changing trajectory. Indirectly modifying the kinetic energy, reducing it, involved in the athlete's run, will positively act on the risk of injuries. In literature a decrement of the kinetic energy up to 3% in steep terrain when used with longer skis, that had a lower standing height and width, was reported. Higher values, up to 7%, could be reached if the effect of snow friction coefficient was considered [5, 6].

Higher jump trajectories lead to create a greater strength that causes imbalance to the back of the trunk. This air resistance increases even more at high speeds. When a slope is designed, the first target must be to reduce the risk of injury: limit the maximum flight's height and conceive the previous part of the track so as not to reach high speeds that favor asymmetrical positions [7]. A jump along the slope could be simulated to predict the jump flight phase. The takeoff inclination and the approaching speed were the main parameters on which to act on to reduce the maximum height of the jump. The weather conditions must always be considered, especially the wind because it could alter the phase of flight. It was possible also to change the curvature of the landing surface to make the landing safer [8].

Knee sprains with the involvement of anterior cruciate ligament (ACL) were one of the most common injuries in skiers. It was reported that aggressive ski behavior was involved in ACL injuries. It was a mechanical situation in which the skier couldn't get off the edge of the ski while it's carving due to an extreme force relationship with the snow. In those situations where the skier's balance was suddenly changed, if there was this phenomenon, the ski control could become unpredictable favoring ACL injury mechanisms. Studies were performed to develop new materials and choose their best features. In GS was reported that higher sidecut radius, 35 and 40 meters (m), compared with 27 m, let to a lower perception of the skis' aggressiveness and force relationship with the snow. Only with the 40 m the external attractiveness was found decreased [6, 9].

The International Ski Federation (FIS) changed the ski regulations for the beginning of the 2012/2013 season. The ski length and the sidecut radius were changed, increasing them, in DH, SG, and SL (Fig. 11.1). The biggest change was made in SG where the sidecut radius moved from 27 to 35 in men and from 23 to 30 in women. It was investigated whether these changes have had an impact on the incidence of injuries in the following seasons. The absolute injury rate, reported for every 100 athletes in every season, in the three seasons after the new ski FIS rules were adopted, was less than the six seasons before. Nevertheless the rate of knee injuries was unchanged as well as that of the lower limbs. The lower number of

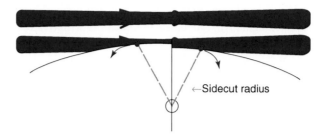

Fig. 11.1 Two different hypothetical sidecut radii and their effect on the ski shape. The sidecut radius on the left is greater than of the right one

injuries was due to the lower number of falls and therefore injuries to the upper limbs. Modifications of FIS rules lead to direct and indirect effects immediately, but their long-term actions will be observed after several seasons [10].

However, it is essential that we always continue to work to new ideas, suggestions, and changes to the FIS rules, not stopping to those just introduced. This can be done without forgetting the past and, at the same time, always looking to the future.

An increased sidecut radius in GS reduced the kinetic energy up to 5.6%, but it was mainly due to the different mechanism of turning. A reduction of kinetic energy and therefore the speed may lead to a lower risk of injuries, but this advantage of using this type of skis wasn't so obvious if we consider injuries in the falls or crashes [11].

A greater sidecut radius reduced the self-steering effect of the ski which was a key element in mechanism of ACL injury in alpine ski. The self-steering effect usually makes the athletes unable (or less able) to control the skis [12].

There were skis with different waist widths, from 65 millimeters (mm) to 110 mm, went through 88 mm. Everyone of these lead skiers to a different biomechanical style of skiing. Icy snow tackled with large waist skis increased the risk of degenerative knee injuries because the biomechanics of the skiing brought the knee to extreme movements. External rotation of the knee was increased with the use of wide skis. On the other side, narrow skis lead to an increased knee abduction [13].

FIS regulated in slalom only the minimal waist width of the skis, which must be greater than and/or equal to 63 mm, but it didn't do the same for the maximum waist width, like it did in the other race's categories. This could be a point on which FIS could act in the future to prevent injuries, especially on icy snow [14].

Course setting itself had a role in injury prevention and speed control. Indeed International Ski Federation (FIS) had rules for course length, difference in altitude, and setting [6, 15].

Rules must be chosen carefully. It was reported that increasing horizontal distance between the gates reduces athlete's speed, but on the other hand, this modification to the track could give rise to fatigue early and increase the risk of unbalance in the turns [16].

Small bumps were reported to be one of the most important contributors to the imbalance of the athletes and to ACL injury mechanisms [17].

Aggressive and icy snow were reported to be a risk factor for the slip-catch ACL injury mechanism. However the most contributive element to knee injuries is the presence of snow conditions which change down the track [17].

The impact of snow characteristics was noted in recent studies in which the presence of a fresh snowfall significantly reduced the severity of injuries, based on the ISS [18, 19].

Injected snow and icy conditions were considered less risky by the experts, but a key element in reducing the number of injuries was the uniformity of the snow characteristics along the entire slope [4].

Gates are part of the track to trace the course. In races, the paths chosen by the athletes and the technical approach to the gates are all elements aimed to gain time.

Gates have specific FIS requirements that must be observed in order to reduce the risk of injury. Over the years there was an evolution of the gates. They started from wooden poles to the most recent made of new materials with elastic characteristics that don't produce splinters. Excluding DH, in the other disciplines, gates have a spring joint that bends on when athletes hit the poles, which mustn't leave the snow ground. Further improvements have been made to the panel release system that should release upward from the poles and is now made by a material that breaks down above a specific energy [20].

During the 2006–2009 World Cup (WC) seasons, about 40% of injuries (excluding knee) were involved in the impact with gates, which normally in the technical disciplines (giant slalom and super-G) happens at 60–80 km/h. This causes direct trauma, but we know that it can also act indirectly, unbalance athletes, and get them to fall [20].

The contact with the safety nets or material causes only 10% of the injuries. In all other cases, the assumed time of injury was before the contact with the net.

There are different types of safety nets with different geometries and sizes of the holes. In the past holes were larger than today: it was reported the death of an athlete as a result of injuries suffered in a lower limb stuck in the nets. Other measures are used to improve safety. One of them is to create free spill zones, the space between the race tracks and the nets, because they let the athletes to slip unhindered during a fall.

All safety systems must have the aim to reduce the speed during the fall [20].

There are three types of nets that should be placed along a track. Type A-net is used to avoid falls from high and into ravines. It is fixed to the ground with metal hooks, placed where no other safety system can be used and should not be placed if it avoids a secure spill zone. The net is 4 m high, 25 m long with 5 mm plait, and a 7×7 cm mesh (Fig. 11.2).

Type B-net is a mobile net used to avoid falls from lower height and structure close to the track, like tree lines. It is placed in the snow with 2.5 m high poles, every 2 m, made in PVC (polyvinyl chloride), and usually multiple lines are required, especially on the top of the banks. The net is 2 m high, 15 m long with 3.5 mm plait,

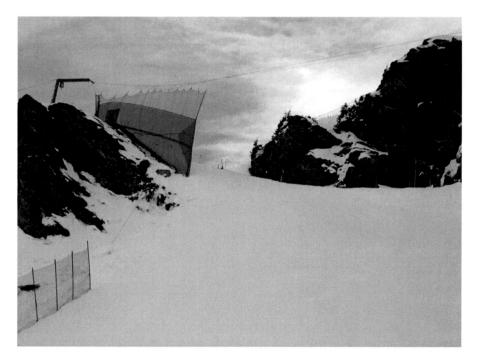

Fig. 11.2 Type A-net

and a 7 × 7 cm mesh. The C-net is placed to avoid outside entry to the track (Fig. 11.3).

When the nets are placed very close to the slope, and therefore to the athlete's trajectory, they may be covered by tarpaulins in order for the athletes to avoid getting stuck in the nets and allow their slippage in the event of accidental impact.

In some cases after a trajectory error, the athletes use this possibility of slipping to not lose the balance, lean on the tarpaulins, and continue their race.

In addition to safety nets, there are other security systems used like the air fence, introduced from motorcycle racing, or like the coloration of the track, made with appropriate signs to highlight the track's limits and jumps or others (Fig. 11.4).

FIS let athletes to use body protectors, but only for forearm and shin can be used over the racing suit. Air bag systems (Dainese) under the suits were tested in alpine ski and started to use in high-velocity disciplines [21].

The helmet must be worn by all athletes during the competitions.

We must always remember that an adequate physical preparation is essential to reduce the risk of injury [4].

If the evolution of materials has led to fewer injuries in adults, a number of injuries in children continued unabated. In children's ski equipment, the problem is that the development is done by adapting adult's materials to children's size, not considering the different characteristics related to age and development. Slope

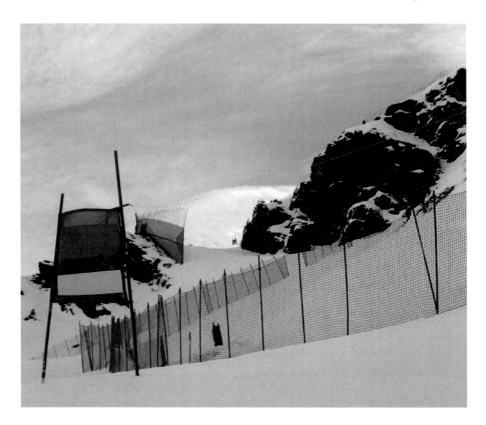

Fig. 11.3 Types B-net and C-net

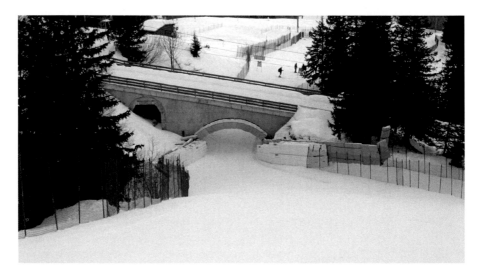

Fig. 11.4 Air fence used to cover cement walls

and snow characteristics were involved equally both in the minor and in severe injuries [22].

11.1 FISI: Italian Winter Sports Federation's Experience

In the last years, the international ski's teams understood the importance of epidemiological data collection of the injuries during the season. Data are used to prevent accidents in races and trainings and to improve athletic training with specific exercises. It must act on two different levels of prevention, active and passive. The FISI, Italian Winter Sports Federation, recorded athlete's injuries since 1985. Until 2009, in 25 years, the population is made of around 600 athletes, and around 850 injuries were recorded.

The fractures account only 14% of all injuries and sprain traumas (54%) were the most frequent. Contusions (8%) and neurological injuries (6%, like concussion) were less common. Spine traumas, muscles injuries, wounds, dislocations, and other injuries together account only the 18% of all.

Considering the frequency of injuries according to anatomical localization, the knee is the most frequently involved, with 52%. It was followed by the ankle (9%), head (9%), trunk (8%), leg (6%), shoulder (6%), thigh (3%), hand (3%), and others (4%).

If the injury affects the upper limb, the shoulder is involved in over half the cases (51%). In the last years, the involvement of the hand and wrist up to 28% of the injuries of the upper limb was increased.

On the other hand, the knee is the anatomical region most affected in the injuries of the lower limb (72%).

In 2009 the incidence of ACL injuries per 1000 hours of activity (training and race) in the skiers was calculated (Table 11.1). In the same study, it was seen that the incidence of ACL injuries in Alpine Ski was, in that period, higher than in football (data from FIGC, Federazione Italiana Giuoco Calcio—Italian Football Federation) and lower than in rugby (data from FIR, Federazione Italiana Rugby—Italian Rugby Federation).

In the 2010/2011 season, we had a total of 32 injuries in 71 alpine skiing FIS athletes. There were 14 sprains, 7 fractures, 6 contusions, and 5 miscellaneous injuries (e.g., tendinopathy, etc.). The knee was involved in half of the injuries: seven

Table 11.1 FISI's injuries data in the season 2006–2009

	Ski	Snowboard
Athletes	150	25
Total injuries in the last 4 years	140	47
Total injuries incidence	0.23	0.45
ACL injuries incidence	0.023	0.013
Upper limb injuries incidence	0.017	0.14

Incidence is calculated per 1000 h of activity

Table 11.2 Injuries divided by anatomical region in two seasons 2010/2011 (71 alpine skiing FIS athletes) and 2012/2013 (70 alpine skiing FIS athletes)

Anatomical region	Injuries (season 2010/2011)	Injuries (season 2012/2013)
Head	0	1
Neck	1	0
Chest/abdomen	1	1
Back	2	6
Shoulder	0	3
Wrist/hand	5	3
Hip	2	0
Thigh	2	0
Knee	16	17
Lower leg	3	2

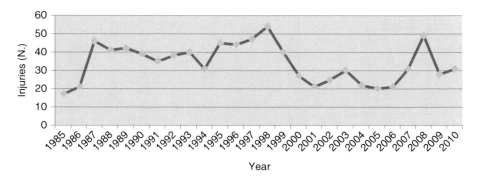

Fig. 11.5 Number of injuries by year of the FISI's ski athletes from 1985 to 2010

isolated ACL injuries, two ACL injuries associated with meniscal lesions, and one isolated meniscal lesion (Table 11.2).

In the season 2012/2013, we had a total of 33 injuries in 70 alpine skiing FIS athletes. There were 14 sprains, 5 fractures, 4 contusions, and 10 miscellaneous injuries. There was an increase incidence, six cases, in injuries of the back. The knee was involved 17 times: five isolated ACL injuries, two isolated meniscal lesions, one ACL and medial collateral ligament (MCL) associated injury, and one osteochondral lesion (Table 11.2).

The ski equipment changes do not always lead to an immediate reduction in the number of injuries. In the FISI's database, it was seen that in the 1990s with the modification of the skis, in the first period, an increase in the number of injuries has been found. This number decreased in a few years, up to values lower than the beginning, thanks to the adaptation of athletes to the new materials, to changes in training techniques and subsequent modifications of the materials themselves. It is essential to monitor injuries both short and long term (Fig. 11.5).

Our data are similar with those of other studies on populations of World Cup skiers reported in the literature and in international conferences.

References

1. Hébert-Losier K, Supej M, Holmberg HC (2014) Biomechanical factors influencing the performance of elite alpine ski racers. Sports Med 44(4):519–533
2. Burtscher M, Ruedl G (2015) Favourable changes of the risk-benefit ratio in alpine skiing. Int J Environ Res Public Health 12(6):6092–6097
3. Klous M, Müller E, Schwameder H (2012) Three-dimensional knee joint loading in alpine skiing: a comparison between a carved and a skidded turn. J Appl Biomech 28(6):655–664
4. Spörri J, Kröll J, Amesberger G, Blake OM, Müller E (2012) Perceived key injury risk factors in World Cup alpine ski racing—an explorative qualitative study with expert stakeholders. Br J Sports Med 46(15):1059–1064
5. Gilgien M, Spörri J, Kröll J, Müller E (2016) Effect of ski geometry and standing height on kinetic energy: equipment designed to reduce risk of severe traumatic injuries in alpine downhill ski racing. Br J Sports Med 50(1):8–13
6. Müller E, Spörri J, Kröll J, Hörterer H (2016) Equipment designed to reduce risk of severe traumatic injuries in alpine ski racing: constructive collaboration between the International Ski Federation, industry and science. Br J Sports Med 50(1):1–2
7. Heinrich D, van den Bogert AJ, Nachbauer W (2014) Relationship between jump landing kinematics and peak ACL force during a jump in downhill skiing: a simulation study. Scand J Med Sci Sports 24(3):e180–e187
8. Schindelwig K, Reichl W, Kaps P, Mössner M, Nachbauer W (2015) Safety assessment of jumps in ski racing. Scand J Med Sci Sports 25(6):797–805
9. Kröll J, Spörri J, Gilgien M, Schwameder H, Müller E (2016) Effect of ski geometry on aggressive ski behaviour and visual aesthetics: equipment designed to reduce risk of severe traumatic knee injuries in alpine giant slalom ski racing. Br J Sports Med 50(1):20–25
10. Haaland B, Steenstrup SE, Bere T, Bahr R, Nordsletten L (2016) Injury rate and injury patterns in FIS World Cup Alpine skiing (2006–2015): have the new ski regulations made an impact? Br J Sports Med 50(1):32–36
11. Kröll J, Spörri J, Gilgien M, Schwameder H, Müller E (2016) Sidecut radius and kinetic energy: equipment designed to reduce risk of severe traumatic knee injuries in alpine giant slalom ski racing. Br J Sports Med 50(1):26–31
12. Spörri J, Kröll J, Gilgien M, Müller E (2016) Sidecut radius and the mechanics of turning-equipment designed to reduce risk of severe traumatic knee injuries in alpine giant slalom ski racing. Br J Sports Med 50(1):14–19
13. Zorko M, Nemec B, Babič J, Lešnik B, Supej M (2015) The waist width of skis influences the kinematics of the knee joint in alpine skiing. J Sports Sci Med 14(3):606–619
14. Supej M, Senner V, Petrone N, Holmberg HC (2017) Reducing the risks for traumatic and overuse injury among competitive alpine skiers. Br J Sports Med 51(1):1–2
15. Gilgien M, Crivelli P, Spörri J, Kröll J, Müller E (2015) Characterization of course and terrain and their effect on skier speed in World Cup alpine ski racing. PLoS One 10(3):e0118119
16. Spörri J, Kröll J, Schwameder H, Schiefermüller C, Müller E (2012) Course setting and selected biomechanical variables related to injury risk in alpine ski racing: an explorative case study. Br J Sports Med 46(15):1072–1077
17. Bere T, Flørenes TW, Krosshaug T, Nordsletten L, Bahr R (2011) Events leading to anterior cruciate ligament injury in World Cup Alpine Skiing: a systematic video analysis of 20 cases. Br J Sports Med 45(16):1294–1302
18. Moore SJ, Knerl D (2013) Let it snow: how snowfall and injury mechanism affect ski and snowboard injuries in Vail, Colorado, 2011–2012. J Trauma Acute Care Surg 75(2):334–338
19. Girardi P, Braggion M, Sacco G, De Giorgi F, Corra S (2010) Factors affecting injury severity among recreational skiers and snowboarders: an epidemiology study. Knee Surg Sports Traumatol Arthrosc 18(12):1804–1809

20. Bere T, Flørenes TW, Krosshaug T, Haugen P, Svandal I, Nordsletten L, Bahr R (2014) A systematic video analysis of 69 injury cases in World Cup alpine skiing. Scand J Med Sci Sports 24(4):667–677
21. Dainese (2012) D-air@ Protection [online] [cited 2012 Jan 25]. http://www.dainese.com/eu_en/d-air/d-air-racing
22. Meyers MC, Laurent CM Jr, Higgins RW, Skelly WA (2007) Downhill ski injuries in children and adolescents. Sports Med 37(6):485–499

Chapter 12
Respiratory System Illness and Hypoxia

Manuela Bartesaghi and Giuseppe Miserocchi

Abstract Exposure to hypobaric hypoxia results in a reduction of the passage of O_2 from the alveoli to the blood, reducing the amount of circulating oxygen and requires physical adaptations and physiological changes in every people.

The duration and degree of hypoxic exposure are critical to the metabolic response of skeletal muscle, with the response to acute hypoxia during exercise. Many changes in the pathways of oxygen delivery have been characterized in hypoxic humans at real or simulated altitude. In contrast, relatively little is understood about changes in tissue oxygen utilization in humans at altitude.

12.1 Hypobaric Hypoxia

During flights at high altitude or mountain climbing, people are subjected to the effect of reduced air pressure and, consequently, to lower partial pressure of O_2. The concentration of oxygen in air remains constant so, as the barometric pressure decreases, the partial pressure of oxygen decreases proportionately, challenging oxygen delivery to the tissues. This condition is referred to as hypobaric hypoxia.

Exposure to hypobaric hypoxia results in a reduction of the passage of O_2 from the alveoli to the blood, reducing the amount of circulating oxygen.

The exposition to high altitude requires physical adaptations and physiological changes in every people.

The positive aspects of high-altitude acclimatization, most notably decreased susceptibility to acute mountain sickness, also contrast with the less well-understood phenomenon of high-altitude deterioration, which occurs with prolonged exposure

M. Bartesaghi (✉)
Italian Winter Sports Federation, Milano, Italy

Ambulatory of Clinic Physiology and Sport, University of Medicine Milan-Bicocca,
Via Cadore 48, 20900 Monza, Italy
e-mail: Manuela.bartesaghi@outlook.it

Ambulatory of Sport Medicine, Pentavis, Via Carlo Cattaneo 69, Lecco, Italy

G. Miserocchi
Ambulatory of Clinic Physiology and Sport, University of Medicine Milan-Bicocca,
Via Cadore 48, 20900 Monza, Italy

© Springer International Publishing AG 2018
H. Schoenhuber et al. (eds.), *Alpine Skiing Injuries*, Sports and Traumatology,
https://doi.org/10.1007/978-3-319-61355-0_12

to extreme high altitude (>5500 m) and is characterized by lethargy, fatigue and muscle wasting [1–9].

High-altitude physiology may be divided into short-term changes that occur with exposure to hypobaric hypoxia (the acute response to hypoxia) and longer-term acclimatisation and adaptation. Acute exposure to the ambient atmosphere at extreme altitude (e.g., above 8000 m) is rapidly fatal [10]. Acclimatisation is the set of beneficial processes whereby lowland humans respond to a reduced inspired partial pressure of oxygen, and it begins already at 2500 m above sea. These changes tend to reduce the gradient of oxygen partial pressure from ambient air to tissues (classical oxygen cascade) and are distinct from the pathological changes that lead to altitude illness. High-altitude illness may be divided into the acute syndromes (AMS) that affect lowland ascending to altitudes and the chronic conditions that affect individual resident at high altitude for long periods. The AMS, if not recognized and treated, could degenerate into high-altitude pulmonary oedema (HAPE) and high-altitude cerebral oedema (HACE).

The incidence and severity of acute mountain sickness, HAPE, and HACE are related to the speed of ascent and the maximum height gained, suggesting a dose–response type of relationship in susceptible individuals [2]. A number of studies also suggest, however, that inflammation may be contributory in the pathogenesis of altitude illness [2].

The physiological response to acute hypobaric hypoxia serves to increase oxygen delivery to the tissues: ventilation, cardiac output and haemoglobin concentrations increase (haemoglobin concentration increases initially by the haemoconcentration and later as a result of increased erythropoiesis). Similarly, the textbook paradigm of acclimatisation to hypobaric hypoxia emphasises the development of mechanisms to increase oxygen flux (increase in ventilation, cardiac output, oxygen carriage and capillarity) [10].

These observations, however, do not adequately explain the observed differences between individuals in their tolerance of hypobaric hypoxic environments. Neither the baseline cardiorespiratory performance (maximal oxygen consumption) nor changes in the response to chronic hypoxia account for differences between individuals in acclimatisation to prolonged hypoxia [3] or performance at altitude [4]. Maximal oxygen consumption, maximal heart rate and stroke volume are all reduced [5] after acclimatisation despite normalisation of the blood oxygen content to sea-level values (by an increase in haemoglobin concentration) [6]. Furthermore, pure oxygen breathing by acclimatised individuals (which results in an oxygen content greater than that at sea level) does not return maximal oxygen consumption to sea-level values [7]. These surprising findings suggest that oxygen carriage is not a limiting factor for maximal oxygen consumption at altitude. This could be consistent with central nervous system limitation of the maximal exercise capacity, with limitation of oxygen flux within the tissues or with a downregulation of cellular metabolism [10].

An alternative model supported by empirical evidence suggests that mechanisms not related to oxygen delivery may play an even greater role: this alternative model proposes that acclimatisation is achieved not solely by increasing the oxygen flux but also by decreasing utilisation. Acclimatisation may therefore be mediated in part by alterations in oxygen delivery, but also by reductions in cellular oxygen demand, perhaps through hibernation/stunning or preconditioning pathways or through improvements in efficiency of use of metabolic substrates.

Hypoxia is not, however, the only stress encountered at altitude. Temperature falls with increasing elevation, whilst absolute humidity is extremely low and exposure to solar/ultraviolet radiation high. Visitors frequently experience gastrointestinal upset and appetite loss, which could result from the hypoxia itself, but may be exacerbated by infection, particularly in developing countries [11]. In addition, activity levels are often altered, as oxygen delivery limits exercise capacity and motivation falls; thus, individuals may undergo detraining [12].

12.2 Hypobaric Hypoxia and Exercise in Alpine Sky

In some period of training, also Italian skiing team is exposed to high altitude. Indeed, in the USA, many sky resorts provide access to mountain as high as 3050–4270 m. During the USA transfers in November (usually in Colorado), athletes stay for more than 2 weeks around 3000 m.

The duration and degree of hypoxic exposure are critical to the metabolic response of skeletal muscle, with the response to acute hypoxia during exercise or relatively [8].

Many changes in the pathways of oxygen delivery have been characterized in hypoxic humans at real or simulated altitude. In contrast, relatively little is understood about changes in tissue oxygen utilization in humans at altitude [13, 14].

Tissue hypoxia may be due to decreased tissue oxygen delivery associated with microcirculatory dysfunction or may occur via alterations in cellular energy pathways and mitochondrial function, resulting in a decreased ability to utilise the available oxygen [12].

In hypobaric hypoxia, mitochondrial respiration and aerobic capacity are thus limited, whilst reactive oxygen species (ROS) production increases [15].

Skeletal muscle, like all oxidative tissues of the body, is critically dependent on a supply of oxygen to maintain energetic and redox homeostasis. ATP can be synthesised in the skeletal muscle in an oxygen-dependent manner in the mitochondria via oxidative phosphorylation, utilising substrates such as glycolytically derived pyruvate, fatty acids, amino acids and ketone bodies, but also in an oxygen-independent manner in the cytosol, via glycolysis with the resulting pyruvate converted to lactate [16].

At moderate high altitude, even with prolonged exposure, no such loss in mitochondrial volume density occurs, although notably, lower muscle mitochondrial densities have been reported [17]. Even if literature describe changes in muscle respiratory function occur also at moderate altitudes, but again this may be dependent on the extent of exposure. Two similar high-resolution respirometry studies by Lundby and co-workers described a loss of respiratory capacity and improved coupling following 28 days at 3454 m, but no changes after 9–11 days at 4559 m [11–14, 18–23].

Despite changes in resting metabolites, however, muscle PCr recovery half-times following an exercise challenge were remarkably well preserved in subjects returning either from Everest Base Camp or the summit, indicating that muscle capacity for ATP synthesis may in fact be spared [19].

Many of the metabolic changes reported in humans at altitude have also been observed in hypoxic cells in culture and are associated with stabilization of the hypoxia-inducible factor (HIF) family of transcription factors [9], which controls the expression of hundreds of survival genes related to energy metabolism.

An alternative possibility to low muscle PO_2 per se could be reactive oxygen species (ROS)-mediated effects, because mitochondrial ROS production increases in hypoxia and is modelled to increase sharply in muscle in altitudes. Reactive oxygen species have sometimes been described as indiscriminate mediators of damage to lipids, protein and DNA, and this may be the case when generated in large quantities, but at more moderate concentrations, they play an important signalling role within the cell and can, for instance, bring about stabilization of HIF-1α. This might suggest that transient production of ROS during training (possibly as a result of acute hypoxia due to high rates of muscle O_2 consumption) may elicit training-induced changes, in agreement with a signalling role. Moreover, as outlined elsewhere in this issue of Experimental Physiology by Lundby [23], the response to hypoxia may in fact mediate some aspects of endurance training in muscle [8].

This is an important factor for not giving oxygen at intermediate altitudes, such as 3000 meters, during aerobic training workouts not maximal, because it may have more disadvantages than advantages.

Indeed restoration of P_{aO2} with supplementary O_2 does not fully restore aerobic capacity in acclimatised individuals, possibly indicating a peripheral impairment [15].

Qualitative changes in mitochondrial function also occur and do so at more moderate high altitudes with shorter periods of exposure. Electron transport chain complexes are downregulated, possibly mitigating the increase in ROS production. Fatty acid oxidation capacity is decreased, and there may be improvements in biochemical coupling at the mitochondrial inner membrane that enhance O_2 efficiency. Creatine kinase expression falls, possibly impairing high-energy phosphate transfer from the mitochondria to myofibrils. In climbers returning from the summit of Everest, cardiac energetic reserve (phosphocreatine/ATP) falls, but skeletal muscle energetics are well preserved, possibly supporting the notion that mitochondrial remodelling is a core feature of acclimatisation to extreme high altitude [15].

At altitude, however, creatine kinase is downregulated, potentially impairing high-energy phosphate transfer [15]. Muscle fibre wasting may mitigate this to some extent, by decreasing average diffusion distances, but it is possible that with a compromised capacity for PCr synthesis, the preferred maintenance of mitochondria in intermyofibrillar regions circumvents some of the resulting limitations of high-energy phosphate delivery to myosin.

Notably, however, protein levels of pyruvate dehydrogenase were also lower in these subjects following ascent of Everest, perhaps arguing against as witch towards glucose oxidation and instead supporting a possible increased role for glycolytic ATP production and lactate production instead, bypassing the mitochondria.

With the downregulation of oxidative enzymes and loss of mitochondrial density, it is conceivable that anaerobic glycolysis might make a greater contribution to muscle ATP demands at extreme altitude, particularly during exercise. In humans, however, the evidence to support increased glycolysis at altitude is limited [21]. Indeed, in muscle biopsies from humans returning from extreme altitude, the levels of several glycolytic enzymes were decreased as was hexokinase activity. These observations might reflect the so-called 'lactate paradox'. In this phenomenon, acute exposure to high altitude is accompanied by greater blood lactate levels ($[La_b]$) at a given submaximal workload than at sea level, although following acclimatisation over a period of weeks, the same exercise challenge results in a lower $[La_b]$, more comparable with that at sea level [8]. Thus, acclimatisation may decrease the initial dependence on glycolysis to meet cellular ATP demand, perhaps through multiple adjustments that optimise O_2 delivery and utilisation or through better coupling of pyruvate production and oxidative phosphorylation. Some studies, however, have suggested that the 'lactate paradox' is a more transient feature of acclimatisation and not applicable to those spending longer durations at extreme altitude [15].

Whilst oxidative processes are selectively downregulated in the skeletal muscle following exposure to environmental hypoxia, in contrast to studies in cultured cells, glycolytic markers appear to remain largely unchanged. It is noteworthy, however, that there has been a distinct lack of direct measurements of glycolytic flux in vivo or ex vivo following hypoxic exposure [16].

Today, the lactate paradox is more commonly defined as the phenomenon in which an acute sojourn at altitude induces an increase in blood lactate accumulation during exercise in the short term, yet this decreases after chronic exposure. However, whilst this may reflect some aspect of metabolic remodelling following hypoxic acclimation, current explanations for this phenomenon remain controversial and probably involve factors beyond the mere capacity for substrate utilisation [24].

Taken together, the literature is not clear on whether a hypoxia-induced substrate switch from fatty acid oxidation to glucose oxidation occurs within the mitochondria of skeletal muscle as it does in the hypoxic rat heart, for instance. Environmental hypoxia does however induce a selective attenuation of whole muscle fatty acid oxidation, whilst glucose uptake is maintained or increased, perhaps to support glycolytic flux in the face of a downregulation of oxidative metabolism, optimising the pathways of ATP synthesis for the hypoxic environment [18].

Metabolism is reprogrammed in response to sustained exposure to hypoxia to increase the capacity for anaerobic metabolism and lower that for fatty acid oxidation, which is less O_2 efficient than glycolysis/pyruvate oxidation [16].

In summary, literature report time-dependent changes in gene and protein expression that appear to underlie the mitochondrial response to subacute and sustained hypobaric hypoxia in human skeletal muscle. Following subacute hypoxia exposure, increased uncoupling may serve to protect the mitochondria, particularly the intermyofibrillar mitochondria, but at the cost of impaired efficiency of ATP synthesis [13].

To facilitate adaptation at high altitude is helpful to follow the traditional guidelines for the high altitude, so to expose gradually to high altitude and once achieved hydrated a lot during the stay (useful antioxidant and energy supplements), promoting quality and healthy foods reducing coffee that interfere with rest and then with sleep, already difficult at altitude [25]. About utility of using supplemental O_2 in between heats to facilitate recovery, literature is very discordant and needs further investigations to be able to say with certainty of its usefulness, which at the moment remains doubtful.

Athletes sojourning to high altitude for ski camps can train on immediate ascent but should slowly increase training volume over the first 3 days. Athletes should expect improvements in balance and reaction time 3–6 days into acclimatization. Coaches and athletes should expect about 20% of youth lowlander athletes to have signs and symptoms of AMS during the first 3 days of altitude exposure for alpine lift access sports at altitudes of up to 3800 m [26].

References

1. Hill AB (1965) The environment and disease: association or causation? Proc R Soc Med 58:295–300
2. Hackett PH, Roach RC (2001) High-altitude illness. N Engl J Med 345:107–114
3. Cymerman A, Reeves JT, Sutton JR, Rock PB, Groves BM, Malconian MK, Young PM, Wagner PD, Houston CS (1989) Operation Everest II: maximal oxygen uptake at extreme altitude. J Appl Physiol 66:2446–2453
4. Howald H, Hoppeler H (2003) Performing at extreme altitude: muscle cellular and subcellular adaptations. Eur J Appl Physiol 90:360–364
5. Sutton JR, Reeves JT, Groves BM, Wagner PD, Alexander JK, Hultgren HN, Cymerman A, Houston CS (1992) Oxygen transport and cardiovascular function at extreme altitude: lessons from operation Everest II. Int J Sports Med 13(Suppl 1):S13–S18
6. Calbet JA, Boushel R, Radegran G, Sondergaard H, Wagner PD, Saltin B (2003) Why is VO₂ max after altitude acclimatization still reduced despite normalization of arterial O_2 content? Am J Physiol Regul Integr Comp Physiol 284:R304–R316
7. Cerretelli P (1976) Limiting factors to oxygen transport on Mount Everest. J Appl Physiol 40:658–667
8. West JB et al (2007) High altitude medicine and physiology. Hodder Arnold, London
9. Murray AJ (2016) Energy metabolism and the high-altitude environment. Exp Physiol 101(1):23–27. Department of Physiology, Development and Neuroscience, University of Cambridge, Cambridge, UK
10. Ward MP, Milledge JS, West JB (2000) High altitude medicine and physiology. Arnold, London
11. Margaria R, Edwards HT, Dill DB (1933) The possible mechanisms of contracting and paying the oxygen debt and the role of lactic acid in muscular contraction. Am J Physiol 106:689–715
12. Grocott M (2007) Review: high-altitude physiology and pathophysiology: implications and relevance for intensive care medicine. FASEB J, Crit Care 11(1):203

13. Levett DZ, Radford EJ, Grocott W (2012) Acclimatization of skeletal muscle mitochondria to high-altitude hypoxia during an ascent of Everest. FASEB J 26:1431–1441. www.fasebj.org
14. Murray, A. J. (2009) Metabolic adaptation of skeletal muscle to high altitude hypoxia: how new technologies could resolve the controversies. Genome Medicine 1:117
15. Murray AJ, Horscroft JA (2016) Mitochondrial function at extreme high altitude. J Physiol 594(5):1137–1149. Department of Physiology, Development & Neuroscience, University of Cambridge, Downing Street, Cambridge CB2 3EG, UK
16. Horscroft JA, Murray AJ (2014) Skeletal muscle energy metabolism in environmental hypoxia: climbing towards consensus. Extrem Physiol Med 3:19
17. Kayser B et al (1996) Muscle ultrastructure and biochemistry of lowland Tibetans. J Appl Physiol 81(1):419–425
18. Horscroft JA, Burgess SL, Hu Y, Murray AJ (2015) Altered oxygen utilisation in rat left ventricle and soleus after 14 days, but not 2 days, of environmental hypoxia. PLoS One 10(9):e0138564
19. Edwards LM, Murray AJ, Tyler DJ, Kemp GJ, Grocott CJ, Clarke K, Caudwell Xtreme Everest Research Group (2010) The effect of high-altitude on human skeletal muscle energetics: P-MRS results from the Caudwell Xtreme Everest expedition. PLoS One 5:e10681. https://doi.org/10.1371/journal.pone.0010681
20. Gladden LB (2004) Lactate metabolism: a new paradigm for the third millennium. J Physiol 558:5–30
21. Horscroft JA, Murray AJ (2014) Skeletal muscle energy metabolism in environmental hypoxia: climbing towards consensus. Extrem Physiol Med 3:19
22. Jacobs RA, Boushel R, Wright-Paradis C, Calbet JA, Robach P et al (2013) Mitochondrial function in human skeletal muscle following high-altitude exposure. Exp Physiol 98:245–255
23. Jacobs RA, Siebenmann C, Hug M, Toigo M, Meinild AK et al (2012) Twenty-eight days at 3454-m altitude diminishes respiratory capacity but enhances efficiency in human skeletal muscle mitochondria. FASEB J 26:5192–5200
24. Noakes TD (2009) Last word on viewpoint: evidence that reduced skeletal muscle recruitment explains the lactate paradox during exercise at high altitude. J Appl Physiol (1985) 106:745
25. Chapman RF, Stickford JL, Levine BD (2010) Altitude training considerations for the winter sport athlete. Exp Physiol 95(3):411–421
26. Hydren JR, Kraemer WJ, Volek JS, Dunn-Lewis C, Comstock BA, Szivak TK, Hooper DR, Denegar CR, Maresh CM (2013) Performance changes during a weeklong high-altitude alpine ski-racing training camp in lowlander young athletes. J Strength Cond Res 27(4):924–937